D1116508

A Collection
of Near-Death
Research Readings

A Collection of Near-Death Research Readings

Compiled by

Craig R. Lundahl

Nelson-Hall Publishers nh Chicago

LIBRARY OF CONGRESS CATALOGING IN PUBLICATION DATA

Main entry under title:

A Collection of near-death research readings.

    1. Death—Psychological aspects. 2. Death,
Apparent. I. Lundahl, Craig R.
BF789.D4C64   1982   155.9′37   82-14134
ISBN 0-88229-640-X

Manufactured in the United States of America

10 9 8 7 6 5 4 3 2 1

The paper in this book is pH neutral (acid-free).

CONTRIBUTORS

JOHN R. AUDETTE, M.S., health planning associate, Illinois Central Health Systems Agency; part-time faculty member, Illinois Central College.

K.W.G. BROWN, M.D., associate professor of medicine, University of Toronto.

STEPHEN FRANKLIN, A.B., Cromwell, Connecticut.

CHARLES A. GARFIELD, Ph.D., founder and director, Shanti Project, and assistant clinical professor, Cancer Research Institute, University of California, San Francisco.

MICHAEL GROSSO, Ph.D., assistant professor of philosophy, Jersey City State College.

ERLENDUR HARALDSSON, Ph.D., associate professor of psychology, University of Iceland.

ROY KLETTI, M.A., clinical psychologist, Manitowoc County Counseling Center, Manitowoc, Wisconsin.

SARAH SLOAN KREUTZIGER, M.S.W., assistant professor of social work in psychiatry, University of Florida.

CRAIG R. LUNDAHL, Ph.D., director of research and associate professor of sociology, Western New Mexico University.

R.L. MACMILLAN, M.D., professor of medicine, University of Toronto.

RAYMOND A. MOODY, JR., Ph.D., M.D., Charlottesville, Virginia.

RUSSELL NOYES, Jr., M.D., professor of psychiatry, University of Iowa.

KARLIS OSIS, Ph.D., C.F. Carlson Research Fellow, American Society for Psychical Research.

KENNETH RING, Ph.D., professor of psychology, University of Connecticut.

MICHAEL B. SABOM, M.D., Department of Cardiology, Veterans Administration Hospital, Decatur, Georgia.

HAROLD A. WIDDISON, Ph.D., assistant professor of sociology, Northern Arizona University.

CONTENTS

FOREWORD

DURING THE PAST SEVERAL YEARS, the profound spiritual experiences of persons who come close to death but are reprieved have received attention all over the world. However, as is shown by John Audette's article in the present volume, near-death experiences are definitely not novel events; records of isolated instances go far back into the history of man. One thing which is new, however, is the advent of a modern medical technology which is allowing an ever-increasing number of people to live useful lives after an apparent clinical "death"—or, in more precise terms, a cardiac arrest. It is interesting that so many of these patients return with reports of events which were to them indicative of a life transcending death.

These experiences—especially in the light of the fact that they are, in the great majority of cases, so similar—invite serious considera-tion and reflection. For, even though they do not yield scientific evidence of a life after death, they do suggest profound questions about the nature of the human mind. That is why I am so pleased to see this collection of articles on the subject of the experience of nearly dying. I hope that readers of my own works on the subject— *Life After Life* and *Reflections on Life After Life*—will find this book a useful addition to what I had to say, this time in other words and from other perspectives than my own.

Raymond A. Moody, Jr., M.D.

ix

INTRODUCTION

WHAT HAPPENS AT DEATH HAS CONCERNED all human beings at one time or another. Karlis Osis and Erlendur Haraldsson have said, in *At the Hour of Death* (1977), that "our destiny at death is probably the most important area of human experience into which we can inquire."

For centuries, men of different cultures have speculated about their destiny at death and have encountered near-death experiences. Today, we are in the midst of a death-awareness movement. The meaning of death in human life has once again emerged as a central concern. In the media, the hospital, the classroom, and the home interest continues in this most ancient but most timely of subjects. This interest has been stimulated in particular by the widely publicized work of Elisabeth Kubler-Ross on death and that of Raymond A. Moody, Jr. on near-death experiences.

In the past, the question of what happens at death was usually within the province of philosophy and its arguments, or religion and its determination of man's relation to and attitude toward dying. Today, however, another possible answer to a part of this question may be found through science. In *The Story of Philosophy,* Will Durant (1961) says:

> Every science begins as philosophy and ends as art; it arises in hypothesis and flows into achievement. Philosophy is hypothetical interpretation of the unknown (as in metaphysics), or of the inexactly

known (as in ethics or political philosophy); it is the front trench in the siege of truth. Science is the captured territory; and behind it are those secure regions in which knowledge and art build our imperfect and marvelous world.

The selections in this book suggest that science is beginning to explore a new territory—the subjective experiences of persons near physical death.

Three fields of study have been concerned with various aspects of death. Research on whether human personality survives physical death has been conducted since the 1880s, and one field of study has contributed in particular to the investigation of this phenomenon. This field, parapsychology, has concerned itself with the investigation of mental and physical paranormal phenomena. Thanatology has dealt with the scientific study of death and dying. It began in the last decade and was pioneered by social, behavioral, and medical scientists who were concerned with the treatment and care of dying people and their families. Circumthanatology, the subject of this book, focuses particularly on the scientific inquiry into an aspect of death known as the near-death experience.

Circumthanatology began primarily in this decade and was pioneered by behavioral and medical scientists seeking to scientifically understand this phenomenon. *A Collection of Near-Death Research Readings* was compiled because of the increasing amount of recent scientific work done in this area which is unknown and/or not readily available to researchers, instructors, students, and interested laymen. Thus, the first purpose of this book is to disseminate information on near-death research. The compiler also hopes to encourage further research and teaching in the area of near-death experiences and to contribute to the reevaluation of our society's orientation toward death and the dying.

The selections for this anthology were made on the basis of three criteria: that they fall within one of two lines of inquiry into the study of near death—near-death experiences or deathbed observations—or have particular relevance for the scientific study of near-death phenomena; that they are recent; and that they are scientifically oriented.

The plan of the book is relatively simple. It is divided into five parts: the first is concerned with the relationship between science and near-death experiences; the second deals with a historical perspective of near-death experiences; the third explores recent scientifically oriented research on near-death experiences; the fourth examines theoretical explanations for near-death experiences; and the fifth looks at current directions in near-death research.

In the first part of the book, Harold A. Widdison explores the reactions of scientists in various disciplines to near-death research and the implications of these reactions for further scientific inquiry. He also attempts to show that near-death research is amenable to scientific investigation.

John R. Audette, in the second part, conceptually defines near-death episodes and experiences and then proceeds to provide a portrait of both from a historical perspective. He discusses several historical accounts of near-death episodes and experiences from antiquity to present-day society.

In the third part of the book, some recorded cases and recent systematic research on near-death experiences are presented. In the first selection, one of the first known published medical case histories of a near-death experience is reported by R.L. MacMillan and K.W.G. Brown.

Russell Noyes, Jr., and Roy Kletti follow with a descriptive analysis of 114 accounts of near-death experiences of persons who, mainly, were survivors of accidents. Noyes and Kletti suggest that the subjective phenomenon experienced during extreme life-threatening danger is the result of a syndrome termed depersonalization. According to them, a person uses psychological defenses for handling imminent death.

Karlis Osis and Erlendur Haraldsson provide an elaborate empirical examination of deathbed observations in the United States and India. In their cross-cultural study, physicians and nurses completed questionnaires and were subsequently interviewed concerning 442 cases in the United States and 435 cases in India. They found that four-fifths of the apparitions appearing to terminal patients involved deceased persons and religious figures, and that three out of four apparitions were experienced as having come to take the patients away to a postmortem existence. They found that medical, psychological, cultural, and demographic factors had little or no influence on these deathbed visions.

In the next selection, Raymond A. Moody, Jr. describes eleven elements common to 150 persons who nearly died, citing from case histories.

The next three studies in this section replicate Moody's study. Kenneth Ring, Michael B. Sabom and Sarah Sloan Kreutziger, and Charles A. Garfield all examine the existence and nature of near-death experiences. Ring's systematic study of 102 near-death survivors supports Moody's study, as does Sabom and Kreutziger's study of 100 hospital patients. Garfield's analysis of 215 cancer patients and 36 intensive-care or coronary-care patients lends varied support for the work of Moody and Osis and Haraldsson. In addition, Sabom and Kreutziger briefly outline several theories offering possible explanations of near-death experiences. Sabom and Kreutziger and Garfield also look at some clinical implications of the near-death experience.

In the next selection, I examine eleven accounts of near-death experiences of Mormons between the years 1838 and 1976. Besides corroborating the work of other researchers of near-death with case histories, some over a century old, the study gives insights into the activities and structures of a perceived other-world. The study also sets out two heretofore unmentioned common events which occurred during the near-death experiences of the eleven Mormons.

In the final selection in part three, Kenneth Ring and Stephen Franklin present the first systematic research on near-death experiences associated with suicide attempts. This selection describes three distinct patterns found in suicide-related near-death experiences and the aftereffects of these experiences.

Michael Grosso, in part four of the book, makes an extensive examination of the near-death experience and evaluates some of the explanations for these experiences.

In the fifth and final selection of this book, I describe the major directions near-death research is taking in this decade.

The study of the subjective experiences of persons near physical death, by behavioral and medical scientists, is just beginning to scratch the surface of a phenomenon whose meaning is not yet clear. No one knows what the future holds for this new scientific endeavor; however, there seems to be a definite potential for significant discoveries that could influence the destiny of all mankind. Just the changes in attitude and behavior of those experiencing near-death are testimony to the fact that these experiences cannot be regarded lightly. Hopefully, other serious scientists will lend their abilities and sustained attention to this rich new field of study.

I would like to express my appreciation to several colleagues for their comments and suggestions in the preparation of this volume. They are: John Audette, Donald Gutierrez, David Powell, Ken Ring, Mike Sabom, James Calvert Scott, and Harold Widdison. I am also indebted to the authors who contributed to the volume and the publishers who gave permission to reprint previously published material.

References

Durant, Will. 1961. *The Story of Philosophy*. New York: Simon and Schuster.
Osis, K., and E. Haraldsson. 1977. *At the Hour of Death*. New York: Avon Books.

PART ONE

Science and Near-Death Experiences

1

Near-Death Experiences and the Unscientific Scientist

Harold A. Widdison

In 1975, RAYMOND MOODY PUBLISHED a book purporting to document cases of individuals who had been declared clinically dead but who had revived and, subsequently, reported some very unusual—yet remarkably similar—experiences. Within weeks of publication, the book had become a best-seller and the subject of numerous debates among both scholars and lay persons. The fact that the book stimulated discussion was not surprising, but the unscientific reaction generated within the scientific community was.

The emotional reaction of many scientists to Moody's book was reminiscent of the struggle which took place before science was liberated from the domination of religion. The struggles of Gallileo and Michaelangelo are classic examples of the way scientific advancement can be inhibited by theological perspective. It took hundreds of years before science, as it is known in the western world, came into its own. Even today many scientists feel that religious activity and scientific activity are incompatible and mutually exclusive. Because near-death experiences have been labeled "religious" by some people, scientists have deemed this area as inappropriate for scientific research. While it is true that many individuals do interpret their experiences within a religious framework, near-death research does not necessitate a theological orientation; indeed, the area would be better explored from a scientific, nontheological perspective.

By definition, science must not be committed to any particular theory or theories so that it can maintain an objective posture and, thereby, be in a position to explain why things are the way they are. Scientists believe that anything and everything can and, indeed, should be subjected to rigorous scientific inquiry. Concepts that at first appear to have great explanatory utility actually may be inadequate and even misleading. Examples of misleading ideas that at one time were assumed to be true include the flatness of the earth, the movement of celestial bodies around the earth, and the pooling of "bad" blood within the circulatory system. Scientists also believe that nothing is so small or so trivial that it should be taken for granted and that the true significance of pure research may not be readily apparent. For example, Anton van Leeuwenhoek first observed microbes in 1676, but nearly 200 years passed before Louis Pasteur and Robert Koch discovered the connection between microbes and disease.

Although claiming and attempting to be objective, scientists are not immune to the influence of their respective cultures. The cultural setting in which a particular scientist functions affects the areas which will be researched, the topics selected within these areas, and even the tools and techniques that will be employed in the research. The history of science reveals the extent to which scientific investigation has been subject to cultural influences, yet many contemporary scientists appear to be unaware of the degree to which their research efforts also may be affected.

This paper will explore the reactions of scientists in various disciplines to near-death research, review the scientific method, and examine the implications of these reactions for future scientific inquiry. Finally, near-death research will be reviewed and an attempt will be made to show that this area is amenable to scientific investigation.

REACTIONS OF SCIENTISTS TO NEAR-DEATH RESEARCH

The following views have been compiled from informal discussions, academic debates, articles appearing in the mass media, and articles appearing in semi-professional journals.

Social scientists familiar with near-death research have pointed out that these reports reflect cultural differences. They propose that the cultural specificity of the reported experiences should give any scientist significant evidence as to the source of the experience. They ask: If the accounts are truly glimpses into another world, why don't all the observers report seeing the same things? For example, a Navajo reports seeing a Great Chief standing in a beautiful field, whereas a Catholic reports seeing the Virgin Mary standing in a great cathedral and a Hindu sees a Death Messenger coming to take him away. Therefore, an examination of near-death accounts gives credence to the concept that the afterlife is a mirror image of and hence the product of the culture of the individual. According to sociologists and anthropologists, an individual is conditioned by his culture, and his near-death experiences result from his culturally induced expectations.

Behavioral scientists, primarily psychologists, have theorized that, if an individual consciously or unconsciously senses the imminence of death and cannot accept the idea that he may cease to exist, he will utilize ego-defense mechanisms in an effort to deny death. Psychologists note that although many individuals have had close encounters with death, relatively few have reported near-death experiences. Why focus on the reports, they ask, of a few individuals who may be "deviant cases in the sample" as proof that death does not terminate all aspects of existence? The behavioral scientists postulate, then, that some people cannot accept the inevitability and finality of their own deaths; therefore, their ego defenses redefine into illusions of immortality the sounds and sensations they experience while seriously ill or dying.

Physical scientists, on the other hand, "know" that life ends at the time of biological death and that nothing survives other than an individual's creations, his historical impact, and others' memories of him. Chemists and physicists suggest that the cells of the brain become excited as an individual approaches death and, in this excited state, the information stored there is recalled. They explain that the brain stores information in the form of electrical impulses; when trauma releases these impulses, the individual experiences hallucinations based on memories of persons, actions, and thoughts stored in the brain. These scientists do not attempt to explain why this trauma-induced excitement produces such consistent phenomena in individuals widely separated by time, space, culture, and philosophical/theological orientation.

Medical scientists' objections to accounts of near-death experiences seem to revolve largely around the issue of when the reactions reported as near-death experiences actually occurred. Until fairly recently, it was assumed death occurred when the heart and lungs stopped functioning, because that is when the rest of the body rapidly begins to deteriorate. However, medical scientists have learned to keep the body from deteriorating during resuscitation attempts. Medical doctors now tend to draw a major distinction between *clinical death,* which is reversible, and *death* which by definition is irreversible. Clinical death refers to the period of time when the heart and lungs are not operative but other organs are still functioning. Medical scientists today reason that near-death experiences are produced by the trauma associated with clinical death and are not therefore glimpses into an afterlife. Some physicians may not deny that the individual who reports a near-death experience is sincere or that his experience was real to him; however, they assert that he misperceives the source of the experience which they claim results from pain, drugs, oxygen deprivation, brain disease, and/or high temperatures. Other physicians hypothesize that many accounts represent the hallucinations of mentally unstable individuals in response to intense trauma and stress. Still others believe that the individual experiences what he has been conditioned to by his religious beliefs and orientation.

The foregoing discussion summarizes the unique ways some scientists in four fields have attempted to explain near-death reports. Although these scientists have proposed differing explanations they do agree on one thing: the explanations suggested by the proponents of near-death research are false. In light of this, perhaps the words of Albert Einstein would not be amiss: "It is possible there exists human emanations which are still unknown to us. Do you remember how electrical currents and 'unseen waves' were laughed at? The knowledge about man is still in its infancy (David and Earle, 1978, p. 37)." This observation by one of the greatest scientists of this or any century should remind researchers that the objective scientist maintains an open mind.

THE SCIENTIFIC METHOD

The scientific method has been developed around a series of postulates which include the following (Sjoberg and Nett, 1968, pp. 23-28; Hempel, 1965, ch. 9):

1. All behavior is naturally determined; every event has a natural antecedent of cause.

2. All objective phenomena are eventually knowable; given adequate time and effort, no objective problem is unsolvable.
3. Nothing is self-evident; truth must be demonstrated objectively.
4. Truth is relevant to the existing state of knowledge.
5. All perceptions are achieved through the senses; all knowledge is derived from sensory impressions.
6. Man can trust his perceptions; memory and reasoning are reliable agents for acquiring information.

These postulates are basic assumptions for all scientific inquiry. A discussion of these postulates and their relationship to near-death research follows.

ASSUMPTIONS OF SCIENCE AND NEAR-DEATH RESEARCH

The preceding section summarized the reactions of some scientists to near-death reports. Now these reactions will be evaluated on the basis of these six postulates.

Postulate 1 states that "all behavior is naturally determined; every event has a natural antecedent or cause." The key word is "naturally" which, for the scientist, refers to biological, chemical, or physiological processes operating in or on the body which are either known or can be determined. The problem here is that the concept "naturally" is subject to both professional bias and the state of scientific knowledge. For example, if I had reported to a gathering of scientists two hundred years ago that I could walk into a dark room and, by passing my hand over a particular spot on the wall, cause the room to become as light as day, many of those "objective" scientists would have questioned my sanity, because what I proposed to do would have violated what was then believed to be "nature." If the scientist really believes that every occurrence has an antecedent which ultimately may be identified, why does he restrict "nature" to the state of existing knowledge? Limiting nature to the present state of knowledge inhibits the progress of science.

Postulate 2 states that "all objective phenomena are eventually knowable; given adequate time and effort, no objective problem is unsolvable." The concept "objective phenomena" is also related to the existing state of scientific technology. In the field of high energy physics, for example, scientists are studying the subparticles of matter and antimatter which cannot be seen directly. Yet, by observing the actions of matter as revealed in cloud chambers and studying the reactions that occur when energy fields are altered, these scientists can draw inferences about the properties of something which they are unable to see. Someday they may even develop the capacity to observe subparticles directly and verify the correctness or incorrectness of these inferences. In the area of near-death research, it is equally true that by observing the actions of the dying and studying their reactions to death through the experiences which they report, scientists can draw inferences about a phenomenon which they are unable to see or experience directly. The reactions of the dying constitute an objective phenomenon that can be classified, analyzed, and recorded. The major reason many scientists avoid research in the area of near-death is because of their assumption—which is debatable—that it falls in the general field of spiritualism and religion.

Postulate 3 states that "Nothing is self-evident; truth must be demonstrated objectively." Scientists should neither accept nor reject a hypothesis without first examining all pertinent information. Yet many have rejected research dealing with near-death because the findings suggest a "spiritual existence" that goes against their personal biases, though not against the cannons of scientific inquiry. Therefore, these scientists suggest it would be more appropriate to direct research toward discovering what social and physical factors stimulate these "hallucinations." They permit themselves to engage in premature closure, that is, they have decided on the "answer" before they have reviewed and evaluated all pertinent data.

Postulate 4 says that "truth is relevant to the existing state of knowledge." Most scientists can accept the idea that new discoveries may completely alter "knowledge" as it is currently understood. However, in an area not defined as "appropriate" for scientific inquiry, they will reject completely the results of any and all research. For some scientists, then, truth is restricted to those areas which they define as appropriate for study. If the research falls outside the "approved" areas, even strict adherence to scientific procedures and techniques cannot legitimize the results. Thus, this postulate would seem to be applicable only if the scientific community has recognized the research area.

Postulate 5 and 6 state, respectively, "All perceptions are achieved through the senses; all knowledge is derived from sensory impressions," and "Man can trust his perceptions; memory and reasoning are reliable agents for acquiring information." These postulates imply that it is the scientist's perceptions that constitute scientific knowledge and that unless he can experience phenomena through his own senses research is not possible. Yet, as previously stated physicists are unable to study directly the properties of submatter but can gain knowledge about it by observing the effect matter has on submatter. It is odd, then, that unobservable phenomena in high-energy physics are considered acceptable for scientific inquiry but that near-death experiences are not. If men "can trust their perceptions," then near-death research should be taken as seriously as research concerning high energy physics.

The foregoing discussion suggests the following:

• Scientists are not immune to the influence of their culture.
• Personal values affect what scientists define as appropriate fields of research.
• Scientists tend to condemn research that does not fit their concept of what is "scientific."
• If technology hasn't progressed far enough scientific research may be inhibited.
• The postulates of science are applied differentially depending upon the acceptability of the research area.

These five points reveal why efforts to conduct scientific research in the area of near-death are difficult, at best. Researchers not only fail to receive support from colleagues, but actually are pressured to abandon such research. Yet, in spite of such resistance, some well-designed research has been conducted. In the following section, some of the better research projects are discussed.

NEAR-DEATH RESEARCH

Reports on near-death experiences are not new. Throughout recorded history, supposedly "dead" individuals have revived and startled others with accounts of what they had experienced. According to Budge (1960), the ancient Egyptian *The Book of the Dead* was written to assist the dying with the transition between life and death. In 800 A.D. the Tibetans recorded accounts of near-death experiences in a book whose purpose was to help the dying know what to expect (Fremantle and Chogyan, 1975). Lundahl (1979) reports that Mormons (members of the Church of Jesus Christ of Latter-Day Saints) have given accounts of near-death experiences virtually from the day the church was established in 1830.

Modern accounts have been written detailing experiences of individuals who "died" and returned to tell about it, but none caught the attention and imagination of the public like Raymond Moody's book, *Life After Life* (1975). This book became a best seller largely because it presented interesting case histories. Drawing from experiences reported to him, Moody attempted to analyze the process of death. His book was intended as a report on his exploratory research and not as an exhaustive study of near-death experiences (1975, pp. 15-16). The purpose of *Life After Life* was to develop a general descriptive profile or model based on the reports of his subjects (1975, p. 21), and he suggested that systematic study be undertaken to test his model (1975, p. 6).

Moody's book has spawned numerous reports, books, movies, and lectures which exploit the current intense interest in the possibility of life after death (Ebon, 1977; Hanley, 1977; Matson, 1975; Wheeler, 1976; Wilkerson, 1977). Scientists have pointed to such opportunistic commercializations as evidence of the unscientific nature of the subject. Further, they contend that some people may be reporting experiences they have not actually had. They suggest that impressionable individuals seeking assurance of immortality may accept these accounts as "proof" of life after death and internalize what they have heard or read until they sincerely believe they have had such experiences themselves. Another idea advanced to explain the increasing number of reports suggests the very strong possibility that some persons are seeking to achieve a form of notoriety by claiming to have had "after-death" experiences. The problem facing the researcher, therefore, is to determine the authenticity of these reports.

On the assumption that physicians and nurses are trained to be objective observers of their patients, Osis and Haraldsson (1977) decided to interview medical personnel concerning patients whose deaths they had witnessed. To do this, they mailed questionnaires to 2,500 physicians and 2,500 nurses currently in practice in the United States; they received 1,004 completed questionnaires. Osis and Haraldsson also interviewed 704 physicians and nurses in India. From the 1,708 usable responses, they selected 877 respondents for in-depth interviews. The phenomena reported by the doctors and nurses during these interviews were grouped into the categories of visitation of personages, visions of places, and elevations of mood.

Visitations of Personages

Two-thirds of the sample stated that patients had reported "seeing" a personage before they died, with the majority reporting that they saw deceased rather than living personages. Interestingly, individuals in the hospital who were ill but not terminally so tended to see living personages in their hallucinations, whereas individuals who were terminally ill tended to see deceased personages. Of the deceased personages reported, 91 percent were relatives—usually very close relatives such as mother, father, spouse, offspring, or sibling—of the dying person. The exception to this was the reports of personages who were defined as "religious figures." The exclusive purpose of the personage's visitation was to "take away" the dying patient to another mode of existence. The doctors and nurses reported that the most common reaction to the personage was that of peace, serenity, religious elation, and other-worldly feelings (Osis and Haraldsson, 1977, pp. 56-57).

Visions of Places

The researchers contrasted reports of places and settings of "this world" with reports of places and settings "not of this world." They concluded that the patients whose experiences encompassed objective this-world places and settings seldom experienced peace, serenity, or religious elation, whereas the opposite was true for those patients whose visions involved other worlds, e.g., "heaven" and beautiful gardens. For the latter, a positive emotional response of peace, serenity, or religious elation dominated. Nearly all patients who gave accounts of other-world visions reported that the scene was one of harmony and great beauty (Osis and Haraldsson, 1977, p. 186).

Elevations of Mood

The physicians and nurses reported to Osis and Haraldsson that many patients displayed an elevation in mood shortly before they died. The majority of their patients "were fully conscious, were not running fevers, were not being affected by sedation, and did not suffer from diseases of the brain or other diseases that are considered apt to cause hallucinations or euphoria (Osis and Haraldsson 1977, p. 122)." Some patients who had been unconscious or semiconscious became fully conscious and communicative during the period of mood elevation. Others, such as chronic psychotics and schizophrenics, who had been out of touch with reality, became lucid in conversation and normal in appearance during the period of mood elevation shortly before they died. Patients who had been in great pain or deep depression were reported suddenly to become peaceful and serene. One nurse stated that it was almost as if they had "turned on an inner light (Osis and Haraldsson, 1977, pp. 120-45)."

The researchers were keenly aware that various scientists have proposed alternative explanations for the phenomena they were investigating. In an attempt to evaluate these alternative explanations, Osis and Haraldsson therefore reevaluated their own data and introduced a number of control variables that might explain the relationships they had found. Controls for age, sex, religious orientation, and interviewer bias indicated that these variables did not explain away the incidence or frequency of near-death experiences. Controls for medical, psychological, and cultural factors, the researchers found, were also not significantly related to near-death experiences. However, because Osis and Haraldsson's analysis plays a major role in the reactions of the scientific community to near-death research, it will be discussed here.

Medical Factors

It is well known that hallucinogenic drugs such as morphine and demerol are frequently administered to the dying to mask their pain. Because of this, medical scientists have postulated that the change in mood and the hallucinations the patients experienced were manifestations of these drugs and nothing else. In analyzing their data, Osis and Haraldsson found that only a small minority of the patients who reported deathbed visions had received such drugs. They also discovered that there was no difference in the frequency of near-death experiences between medicated and nonmedicated patients (1977, p. 107).

In looking at the effects of disease, injury, and uremic poisoning the authors noted that "deathbed phenomena suggestive of an afterlife" were not reported more frequently by individuals with brain disturbances (1977, p. 187). In fact, they found that brain disturbances inhibited rather than increased the incidence of near-death phenomena (1977, 188). In addition, when they examined the histories of individuals reporting near-death experiences, they found no difference in frequency between patients with and patients without histories of hallucinating (1977, 188).

In summarizing their results, Osis and Haraldsson stated that they could not find a medical condition or set of conditions that would account for near-death experiences. In fact, they discovered that "medical factors which cripple communication with the external world also cut down on phenomena related to an afterlife (1977, p. 188)." It is possible that some of the individuals who were unable to communicate had also had near-death experiences but were unable (or refused) to relate them (1977, p. 142).

Psychological Factors

Medical scientists state that, under severe stress or intense expectations, an individual could be expected to hallucinate, that is, the individual would "see" what he wanted or needed to see. (For example, the desert traveler who is severely dehydrated begins to hallucinate the presence of water.) However, Osis and Haraldsson found that near-death phenomena were not related to "indices of stress, expectations to die or to recover, or the patient's desire to see a person dear to him" (1977, p. 188). Thus, their findings did not support scientists' contention that psychological stress provides an adequate explanation for near-death experiences. Indeed, some patients were neither under severe stress nor terminally ill; both they and their families expected them to recover. Seeing a deceased personage who came to take them away to the world of the dead, therefore would be contrary to their expectations (1977, p. 86). Some individuals reported that they attempted to resist the efforts of the personage to take them away, for example, "they cried out for help or tried to hide. Such cases can hardly be interpreted as projected wish-fulfillment imagery" (1977, p. 87). Even more supportive of a nonpsychological explanation were those cases where patients contradicted the prognosis of the attending physician and correctly predicted their own deaths (1977, p. 87).

Cultural Factors

To investigate the influence of cultural factors on near-death experiences, Osis and Haraldsson selected samples from two diverse cultures—the United States and India. They discovered both similarities and differences in what the physicians and nurses reported their patients had experienced; however, the similarities far exceeded the differences.

They discovered that many individuals found it very difficult to describe exactly what they had experienced. Those who attempted to share their experiences tended to draw words and examples from their own culture which they believed the listener would understand. The inference is that otherwise it would be extremely difficult for the patients to explain such a unique experience without utilizing the common reference points that a shared culture provides. While culture therefore dictated the words and examples selected to convey the experience, many individuals reported surprise at what they experienced and stated that what they observed did not conform to what they had been taught to expect (Osis and Haraldsson, 1977, p. 190).

The insights provided by Osis and Haraldsson do not support the social scientists' premise that culture is the primary force behind reports of near-death experiences. Any attempt to describe a very unusual experience will be affected by the linguistic tools an individual has available and the degree to which he shares common experiences with his listeners. For example, in attempting to share the visual impact of a beautiful sunset, the vastness of the Grand Canyon, or the delicate hues of a flower, the individual listening must be able to relate to the scene being described. Thus, a person born blind would not be able to visualize those scenes. Likewise, an individual who had spent his entire life north of the Arctic Circle could not understand what living in a jungle would be like. This would be very close to the problem facing individuals who have had a near-death experience. They become very frustrated in their attempts to find words that reflect accurately what was experienced. They have to be satisfied with inexact comparisons which really do not convey the essence of what was witnessed.

Whereas sociologists and anthropologists have hypothesized that the experiences reported are nothing more than a reflection of the culture system of each individual, those engaged in near-death research believe that *it is the attempt to communicate which is affected by culture.* Thus, by affecting the efforts of the individual to communicate, the cultural system tends to distort the experience. The questions to be answered are: Does culture produce the experience or does it attach culturally specific meanings to the experience?

Scientists generally have accepted the assumption as fact that there is no life after death. Any claim of an experience or stated belief to the contrary is dismissed as the product of cultural conditioning. In the case of near-death experiences, social scientists point to the unique cultural aspects of the reports as evidence that they are products of specific cultures. This bias on the part of social scientists tends to blind them to the remarkable similarities in the accounts. These similarities have remained unaffected by time or cultural differences. Perhaps social scientists need to address the research questions: What accounts for the remarkable similarities in near-death reports and why do these reports persist over time and across cultures?

Major advances in technology have opened new vistas in all areas of science. The utilization of particle accelerators has enabled scientists to "crack the atom," create new elements, and analyze the nature of matter. Similarly, the application of high voltage research to the field of photography has resulted in the corona discharge, or Kirlian, technique. This technological advance has implications for near-death investigations.

Kirlian Research

Corona discharge, or Kirlian, photography is based on the action of high voltage currents. Perhaps the best known application of Kirlian photography is the "phantom leaf effect." This effect is produced by taking a leaf with anywhere from 2 to 10 percent of the leaf cut away and photographing it using the Kirlian technique. When the plate is developed, sometimes the image of the entire leaf appears (Davis and Lane 1978, pp. 46-48; Krippner and Rubin, 1974, pp. 60-61, 78). The phrase "phantom leaf effect" refers then to the photographing of the part of the leaf that had been removed and that had not been present when the photograph was actually taken. The phantom leaf effect suggests the possibility that living organisms may be composed both of a biological component (which can be photographed using the conventional technique) and a nonbiological component (which can be photographed only when the Kirlian technique is used).

This technological advance poses some questions that near-death researchers and others should seek to answer: Do living organisms have both a biological and a nonbiological component? If there are two components, must they always coexist or can one component exist without the other? If one can exist only in conjunction with the other, then why does the Kirlian photograph differ from the conventional photograph? If the nonbiological component, or "life force" can function independently of the biological component, can the life force exist separately in another dimension? If there is another dimension which coexists with the physical dimension, then is it possible that, as an individual approaches death, his state of consciousness is altered so that he gains glimpses of that other dimension? In the future, rigorous and systematic research, assisted by new and improved technologies, may reveal answers to these questions. It is hoped that scientists from all disciplines will use their skills and training to explore the area of near-death experiences, which has so much potential significance.

References

Budge, E.A. Wallis. 1960. *The Book of the Dead.* New York: Bell Pub. Co.

Davis, Mikol, and Earle Lane. 1978. *Rainbows of Life.* New York: Harper and Row.

Ebon, Martin. 1977. *The Evidence for Life After Death.* New York: New American Library.

Fremantle, Francesca. Trans. by Chooyan. 1975. *The Tibetan Book of the Dead.* London: Shambhala.

Hanley, Elizabeth. 1977. *Life After Death.* New York: Leisure Books.

Hempel, Carl G. 1965. *Aspects of Scientific Explanation.* New York: Free Press.

Krippner, Stanley, and Daniel Rubin (Eds.). *The Kirlian Aura.* Garden City, N.Y.: Anchor Books.

Lundahl, Craig R. 1979. "Mormon Near-Death Experiences." *Free Inquiry in Creative Sociology* 7:101-4, 107.

Matson, Archie. 1975. *Afterlife.* New York: Harper and Row.

Moody, Raymond A., Jr. 1975. *Life After Life.* New York: Bantom Books.

_____. 1977. *Reflections on Life After Life.* Covington, Ga.: Mockingbird Books.

Osis, Karlis, and Erlendur Haraldsson. 1977. *At the Hour of Death.* New York: Avon Books.

Sjoberg, Gideon, and Roger Nett. 1968. *A Methodology for Social Research.* New York: Harper and Row.

Wilkersons, Ralph. 1977. *Beyond and Back.* New York: Bantom Books.

PART TWO

The History of Near-Death Experiences

2

Historical Perspectives on
Near-Death Episodes and Experiences

John R. Audette

REPORTS OF PARANORMAL PHENOMENA associated with near-death episodes have increasingly captured scientific and public attention in recent years, with the fervor of some new serendipitous discovery. Moody's (1975) now classic work on peak experiences of persons nearing physical death, and comparable findings by Elisabeth Kubler-Ross[1] provided the initial momentum. Popular reaction indicated that some new and astounding insights had been gained regarding the ageless dilemma of human mortality and its ultimate ontological significance.

Amid growing subscription to secular attitudes and the predominate belief in the capabilities of modern science, recent studies of persons surviving near-death episodes have supported the hope that empirical perspectives on the enigma of death may be possible for the first time in human history. For many individuals, these research findings have provided a basis for taking the questions of life after death out of the realm of theological obscurantism and dogma. This is a sentiment which has flourished despite the disclaimers of concerned scientists, Kubler-Ross excluded, who have been quick to identify both the limitations of contemporary empiricism and the presence of alternative explanations.

The writer wishes to thank D.S.W., Mike Gulley, M.D., Raymond Moody, M.D., Louise Moody, and Ken Ring, Ph.D. for their respective contributions to this article. He also wishes to thank those responsible for the body of literature referenced in this article, for without the single contributions of those individual authors there would be no historical perspectives to address.

Modern mainstream science, however, has become revered for its advancement in areas traditionally considered to be the province of religion, i.e., the manipulation of physical death itself and, more recently, exploration of human consciousness during near-death episodes. It is hoped by many that the same scientific wizardry that almost completely eradicated infectious disease and more than doubled human lifespan can also furnish evidence to confirm the theory of human immortality, heretofore a matter of religious faith. There seem to be at least two factors that have prompted this point of view: (1) Current medical technology has achieved the ability to mechanically prolong life indefinitely; rejuvenate the nearly-dead; and revive some of those considered clinically dead; and (2) Scientific technique and methodology now allow for systematic and rigorous analysis of the complex variables in research on the altered states of consciousness ostensibly precipitated by near-death episodes.

A near-death episode occurs when an individual comes very close to physical death, is declared clinically dead, or even merely perceives that death is imminent. Near-death experiences, which sometimes occur during near-death episodes, are altered states of consciousness involving unusual, often mystical visions. Both of these concepts, in historical context, are the focus of this article and will be more fully defined later.

Whatever the absolute significance of near-death research findings, it is erroneous to view near-death experiences as the exclusive product of our era. In fact, the purpose of this article is to demonstrate that near-death episodes and near-death experiences did not emerge solely with the advent of modern medicine. Quite the contrary, such experiences have a long and fascinating historical heritage. They have been with us since before the time of Lazarus. Indeed, what we now have before us may be appropriately referred to as the "Lazarus complex revisited (Hackett, 1972)."

A wise philosopher once said that there is no new knowledge, only new interpretations, insights, and methods of saying what has been said before. Presumably, he was commenting on man's apparent penchant for rediscovering the proverbial wheel, for purchasing the same real estate twice. As Ernest Becker (1973, p. x) has commented, "knowledge is in a state of useless overproduction... strewn all over the place, spoken in a thousand competitive voices. Its insignificant fragments are magnified all out of proportion, while its major and world-historical insights lie around begging for attention."

Interestingly, an inquisitive scholar with basic library skills will find that the literature is bulging with historical examples of near-death experiences. There exists a fascinating collage of return-from-the-dead tales. Some are fictional or mythical in nature, as in Shakespeare's "Romeo and Juliet," Tolstoy's "The Death of Ivan Ilyich," or Edgar Allan Poe's "A Descent into the Maelstrom." Although it is true that fiction sometimes has a basis in fact, this article will be limited to nonfictional accounts, those reported and believed to have occurred prior to the recent popularization of these phenomena.

NEAR-DEATH EPISODES

The near-death episode may be defined as one in which an individual is exposed to and subsequently survives an acute life-threatening situation typically characterized by a loss of consciousness and dangerously unstable vital signs. In some instances, vital signs are altogether absent, i.e., there is no discernable cardiac or respiratory activity. Stated another way, near-death episodes are those in which individuals come extremely close to physical death (as defined by existing medical criteria) and subsequently progress to a more stable condition. Essentially, these episodes involve individuals who have physiologically and/or psychologically faced the prospect of their imminent demise.

Near-death episodes are generally precipitated by severe accident, injury, illness, or disease. There are also a number of disorders which can bring about a death-like state. These include asphyxiation, catalepsy, epilepsy, cerebral anemia, apoplexy, shock, freezing, and near-electrothanasia (being struck by lightning). For the most part, accounts of near-death episodes will be found under the headings of clinical death, temporary death, apparent death, pseudo-death, anabiosis, diagnosis/definition of death, suspended animation, premature burial, and so on.

Moody (1977, pp. 125-26) describes five different types of near-death episodes relevant to this article. All are basically variations on the same theme:

1. A person is gravely ill or injured, even to the point where his physicians give him no chance to live. Nonetheless, he never

undergoes an apparent clinical death and, indeed, goes on to eventually recover.

2. A person is gravely ill or severely injured and, at some point, some of the criteria for clinical death are satisfied. For example, his heart may stop beating and/or he may stop breathing. His doctors may actually believe that he is dead. However, resuscitation procedures are immediately begun, and no one actually pronounces him dead. The resuscitation measures work and he lives.

3. A person is gravely ill or severely injured and, as in (2) above, at some point some of the criteria for clinical death are satisfied. Resuscitation measures are begun but do not seem to work, so they are abandoned. His doctors believe that he is dead and at some point he is actually pronounced dead. The death certificate may even be signed. However, at a later time, even after he has been declared dead, resuscitation measures are resumed for some reason and he is revived.

4. A person is gravely ill or severely injured and at some point some of the criteria for clinical death are satisfied. Resuscitation measures are not even begun because the case seems hopeless. His doctors believe that he is dead and at some point he is actually pronounced dead. The death certificate may even be signed. However, at a later time, even after he has been declared dead, resuscitation measures are begun and he is revived.

5. A person is gravely ill or severly injured and at some point some of the criteria for clinical death are satisfied. Resuscitation measures may or may not be begun, but if they are, they are abandoned, and he is believed or even pronounced dead. At a later time, however, he defies the doctors by 'snapping out of it' spontaneously, without resuscitation measures being used.

Moody (1977, p. 125) also makes reference to a sixth version of the near-death episode: "A person finds himself in a situation in which he could very easily be killed or die, even though he subsequently escapes without injury. He reports having a subjective feeling of certainty that he would be dead very shortly. Yet, against all odds, he lives through the ordeal unharmed." The obvious distinction between near-death episodes of this genre and the five described above relates to the fact that in this instance the threat of death is manifest purely on a psychological level; an individual develops the cognitive conviction and the emotional belief that death is surely about to occur but later finds that bodily injury has somehow been averted.

The near-death episodes dealt with in this article are confined to those that have a physiological basis. This is not to say that episodes and resultant experiences of the sixth type are not worthy of examination; they are simply not the focus of this paper. In actuality, it is worthwhile to note that strictly psychologically oriented incidents have inspired experiences very similar to those reported by persons who were close to death or declared dead in the physical sense (see Noyes, 1971; Noyes, 1972; Noyes and Kletti, 1976).[2]

The historical study of near-death episodes is perhaps best begun with a truly excellent article by A. Keith Mant (1976), in which several cases of misperceived death are discussed. He cites, for example, the work of John Bruhier, a French physician. Bruhier authored an article in 1742 which described fifty-two examples of premature burial and seventy-two incidents of misdiagnosed death. Mant goes on to mention an investigation by Fontenelle in 1834, which recorded forty-six cases of premature burial or misdiagnosis. Reference is also made to an 1845 article by Carré, "De la mort apparente," in which the author describes the cases of forty-six persons who spontaneously regained consciousness while awaiting burial, having already been declared dead. What's more, Mant calls attention to the incredible story of M. François Civille, a Norman who lived in the latter part of the sixteenth century. Mr. Civille was allegedly declared dead, buried, disinterred, and resuscitated a total of three times. Perhaps most interesting of all is the case researched by Professor A. Louis in his article "Lettre sur le certitude des signes de la mort," published in 1752:

> The famous Professor Louis, doyen of French medical jurisprudence, described a curious case of conception whilst apparently dead. A young monk stopped at a house where a young girl was laid out for burial and offered to spend the night in the room where the coffin was placed. He stripped the body during the night and had intercourse with it. The following morning, after he had left, the girl was resuscitated as she was about to be interred, and nine months later she gave birth to a child! [Mant, 1976, 222]

In the *English Malady,* published in 1733, an English physician by the name of Cheyne wrote of a man referred to as Colonel Townsend. Townsend, while under the observation of Cheyne and another physician, entered into a state of so-called suspended animation, of his own volition. It was noted that all cardiac and respiratory activity ceased for thirty minutes whereupon he was left for dead. Townsend, however, subsequently recovered with all faculties intact. There is also the case of Cardinal Archbishop Donnet of Bordeaux who told the French Senate of a personal experience which nearly resulted in premature interment. An article in the *Lancet* of 1866 discusses how the Archbishop was mistakingly pronounced dead by a physician and, though unconscious, was able to hear all of the conversation around him as preparations were made for his funeral. He regained consciousness upon hearing a voice which was extremely familiar to him (Mant, 1976, pp. 221-22).

Misdiagnoses of death have occurred throughout history and were particularly common during the nineteenth century when the topic received considerable attention in the medical journals. (Kastenbaum and Aisenberg, 1976, pp. 112-13). Icard, for example, reported about a dozen cases in which persons were erroneously adjudged dead. In one very rare instance, the individual regained consciousness during the funeral ceremony. Coincidentally, the event was witnessed by several physicians. Tebb, another early researcher, contributed information on 219 alleged cases of persons mistaken for dead: "...149 premature interments that actually occurred, ten cases of dissection while life was not extinct, three cases in which dissection of the living was avoided at the last moment, and even two cases in which consciousness returned to the corpse during the process of embalmment" (Kastenbaum and Aisenberg, 1976, p. 113).

In 1945, under the leadership of Dr. V.A. Negovskii, a team of Russian scientists conducted experiments with fatally wounded soldiers near the front lines. After five to six minutes of recorded clinical death, Negovskii was able to restore full cortical function in several of his subjects. Under certain conditions, where there was a low environmental temperature and rapid onset of death, Negovskii found that he was able to completely restore the functions of the higher components of the central nervous system. In simplistic terms, Negovskii's technique involved the injection of warmed blood mixed with adrenalin and glucose as an intra-arterial transfusion, as opposed to the usual method of intravenous transfusion. His basic hypothesis was that while clinical death is in fact the final stage of dying, it is a state which is reversible in many cases (Negovskii, 1962).

William Brossman, an eighty-year-old retired clothing cutter, was pronounced dead by his physician in the winter of 1952 after a careful examination. The body was transported to a funeral establishment for burial preparation. A short time later, the mortician noticed some reflex and respiratory activity. Brossman was rushed back to the hospital where physicians pronounced him dead once more several hours later (Kaempffert, 1953, p. 76). Langone (1972, p. 18) refers to a study by physicians at Cornell Medical Center of fourteen patients who responded to special treatment after having been declared clinically dead. He also discusses the story of Soviet physicist Lev Landau, who was allegedly revived four times from a state of clinical death brought on by critical injuries sustained during a serious vehicular mishap.

Newsweek magazine carried an article on November 13, 1967 which described the interesting story of U.S. Army Specialist Fourth Class Jacky C. Bayne. It seems that Bayne, while serving with the 196th Light Infantry brigade near Chu Lai, Viet Nam, was critically injured during a mine explosion. Military doctors who attended Bayne found no pulse, no breathing, and no audible heartbeat. External cardiac massage and artificial respiration were applied, to no avail. When an electrocardiograph reading showed no activity, Bayne was declared dead. After several hours, a mortician arrived at a graves-registration unit where the body had been placed. The mortician, in initiating the embalming process, exposed the femoral artery and detected a faint pulse. Bayne was immediately transported to the field hospital whereupon a second resuscitation effort succeeded in reviving him. Bayne recovered and was flown back to the States for further treatment and observation.

In an article by Dlin, Stern, and Poliakoff, the following case was discussed:

> One patient whom I did not get to interview was left for dead after a long period of hopeless attempts at resuscitation. The medical team left. The support systems were stopped. While an aide cleaned up, the patient returned to life. He thought he was in the morgue and that an autopsy had just been performed on him. The patient died a few hours later (1974, p. 63).

The *Augusta Chronicle,* a daily newspaper in Augusta, Georgia, carried two articles within a year of each other, one from the

Associated Press, the other from United Press International, each reporting recent examples of near-death episodes. The AP story made headlines on April 13, 1978. It began: "A woman who was pronounced dead but then gasped for breath on a slab in the county morgue more than an hour later was reported nearly fully recovered Wednesday at Shasta General Hospital," in Redding, California. The case involved a thirty-eight-year-old female who was discovered unconscious in a vacant field. She had apparently ingested barbiturates and alcohol simultaneously in what was believed to be a suicide attempt. The county coroner arrived on the scene and found no pulse, respiration, or other life signs. She was taken to the county morgue where doctors pronounced her dead. The woman later gasped for breath and was resuscitated. Physicians attributed her death-like state to hypothermia, or low body temperature.

The UPI report appeared in the *Chronicle* on January 5, 1979. It was a story about a fourteen-year-old youth who had "drowned" in a car submerged in an icy creek following an accident. The boy was reported to have been underwater for more than fifteen minutes and was without signs of life when first retrieved from the wreckage. Resuscitation measures were employed some time later and succeeded in reviving him. According to the article, he was initially able to communicate only two words: "I died."

Pandey (1971) authored an exceptionally insightful article which identified the need for research into the psychological and emotional dimensions of near-death episodes well before the topic became popular. She observed that "Although consciousness is lost to patients prior to actual clinical death, anecdotal reports show that some recovered patients believed they experienced certain mystical events during that period" (pp. 8-9). She also speculated that the reactions to their experiences of those resuscitated would in large part determine future sociocultural attitudes toward death.

Since the publication of Pandey's article, though probably without relation to it, several studies have been conducted in an effort to probe the basic question posited in her work: What are the psychological and emotional concomitants of near-death episodes and their subsequent manifestations? For the most part, the investigations carried out to date indicate that near-death episodes are sometimes accompanied by simultaneously occurring altered states of awareness, most often highly pleasant if not curiously mystical in nature (e.g., Greyson and Stevenson, 1978; Kubler-Ross, 1975;

Moody, 1975, 1977; Noyes and Kletti, 1976; Ring, 1978; Sabom and Kreutziger, 1977). In a far fewer number of investigations, some researchers claim to have examined cases of unpleasant, if not terrifying, altered states of awareness occurring in conjunction with near-death episodes (e.g., Rawlings, 1978, Garfield 1979). This article is intended to focus, though without bias, on the positive reports since they constitute the bulk of accounts found in the literature.

The paranormal phenomena associated with near-death episodes defy definition by their very nature. For the sake of analysis, they can be collectively referred to as peak experiences, near-death experiences, or altered states of consciousness. These are essentially labels which have been applied for classification purposes. Admittedly, near-death experiences do not lend themselves to operational definition and are a bafflement to many who explore them. Nonetheless, there appear to be recurrent motifs, composite imagery, and a series of sequential events which generally characterize most near-death experiences studied to date.

With these observations in mind, it may be said that near-death experiences refer to altered states of consciousness described by persons who have recovered from such episodes. Tart (1972) defines the altered state of consciousness as "a qualitative alteration in the overall pattern of mental functioning such that the experiencer feels his consciousness is radically different from the way it functions ordinarily." In the case of near-death experiences, altered states of consciousness generally take the form of nonordinary modes of awareness and heightened perceptions ostensibly independent of conventional sensory processes. Experients (persons who report near-death experiences) have been found to report sounds, sensations, visions, images, and events they perceived while unconscious and close to death, if not while clinically dead. As noted earlier, similar reports have been made by persons who merely thought they were going to die but never lost consciousness or suffered any harm.

The prototypical near-death experience, à la Moody (1977, p. 5), is depicted as follows:

> A man is dying and, as he reaches the point of greatest physical distress, he hears himself pronounced dead by his doctor. He begins to hear an uncomfortable noise, a loud ringing or buzzing, and at the same time feels himself moving very rapidly through a long tunnel. After this, he suddenly finds himself outside of his own physical

body, but still in the immediate physical environment, and he sees his own body from a distance as though he is a spectator. He watches the resuscitation attempt from this unusual vantage point and is in a state of emotional upheaval.

After a while, he collects himself and becomes more accustomed to his odd condition. He notices that he still has a "body," but one of a very different nature and with very different powers from the physical body he has left behind. Soon other things begin to happen. Others come to meet and to help him. He glimpses the spirits of relatives and friends who have already died, and a loving warm spirit of a kind he has never encountered before—a being of light—appears before him. This being asks him a question, non-verbally, to make him evaluate his life and helps him along by showing him a panoramic, instantaneous playback of the major events of his life. At some point he finds himself approaching some sort of barrier or border, apparently representing the limit between earthly life and the next life. Yet, he finds that he must go back to the earth, that the time for his death has not yet come. At this point he resists, for by now he is taken up with his experiences in the afterlife and does not want to return. He is overwhelmed by intense feelings of joy, love, and peace. Despite his attitude, though, he somehow reunites with his physical body and lives.

Later he tries to tell others, but he has trouble doing so. In the first place, he can find no human words adequate to describe these unearthly episodes. He also finds that others scoff, so he stops telling other people. Still, the experience affects his life profoundly, especially his views about death and its relationship to life.

Historical perspectives on near-death experiences were first detailed by Moody (1977, pp. 65-77), who attempted to juxtapose reports occurring in or near the present with those purported to have occurred in the distant past. He was able to find evidence of parallels in the writings of Plato (428-348 B.C.) and in the Tibetan *Book of the Dead*, which dates back to the eighth century A.D. After examining these and other examples, Moody posited the following conclusion: "Far from being a new phenomenon, near-death experiences have been with us for a long, long time." D. Scott Rogo (1979) also endeavored to develop historical perspectives on both near-death phenomena and deathbed phenomena, although he focused primarily on the latter.

Noyes and Kletti (1976) may be credited with calling attention to the pioneering work of Albert Heim, a Zurich geology professor, who studied a number of persons who survived acute life-threatening situations during the latter part of the nineteenth century. R.C.A. Hunter (1967, p. 123), however, was perhaps the first scholar to reference Heim's work in an article by Pfister (1930). Heim's study may in fact be the first known attempt to conduct a serious exploration of the psychological and emotional concomitants of near-death episodes. His findings were first presented in 1892 after twenty-five years of research. They revealed that 95 percent of his near-death subjects reported subjective experiences amazingly consistent with one another. More often than not, his subjects depicted death as a highly pleasant process:

> There was no anxiety, no trace of despair, no pain; but rather, calm seriousness, profound acceptance, and a dominant mental quickness and sense of surety. Mental activity became enormous, rising to a hundred-fold velocity or intensity. The relationships of events and their probable outcomes were overviewed with objective clarity. No confusion entered at all. Time became greatly expanded... In many cases there followed a sudden review of the individual's entire past; and finally the person falling often heard beautiful music and fell in a superbly blue heaven containing roseate cloudlets. [Noyes and Kletti, 1976, pp. 46-47][3]

Earlier accounts of near-death experiences appear to be as provocative and fascinating as those taking place in our own time. The story of Admiral Francis Beaufort is one case in point.[4] Beaufort came very close to death during a near-drowning incident as a child in 1795. He fell off a vessel anchored in Portsmouth Harbor and did not know how to swim. Rescue attempts were successful after his body had been submerged for a time. He describes the experience resulted from this incident in the following words:

> All hope fled, all exertion had ceased, a calm feeling of the most perfect tranquility superseded the previous tumultuous sensations— it might be called apathy, certainly not resignation, for drowning no longer appeared to be an evil. I no longer thought of being rescued, nor was I in any bodily pain. On the contrary, my sensations were now of rather a pleasurable cast, partaking of that dull but contented sort of feeling which precedes the sleep produced by fatigue. Though the senses were thus deadened, not so the mind; its activity seemed to be invigorated in a ratio which defies all description, for thought rose after thought with a rapidity of succession that is not only indescribable, but probably inconceivable, by anyone who has not

himself been in a similar situation. The course of these thoughts I can even now in a great measure retrace—the event which had just taken place, the awkwardness that had produced it, the bustle it must have occasioned, the effect it would have on a most affectionate father, and a thousand other circumstances minutely associated with home were the first series of reflection that occurred. They then took a wider range—our last cruise, a former voyage and shipwreck, my school, the progress I had made there and the time I had misspent, and even all my boyish pursuits and adventures. Thus traveling backwards, every past incident of my life seemed to glance across my recollection in retrograde succession; not, however, in mere outline as here stated, but the picture filled up every minute and collateral feature; in short, the whole period of my existence seemed to be placed before me in a kind of panoramic review, and each act of it to be accompanied by a consciousness of right or wrong, or by some reflection on its cause or its consequences; indeed, many trifling events which had been long forgotten, then crossed into my imagination, and with the character of recent familiarity.

While serving in the armed forces during World War I, author Ernest Hemingway was exposed to a life-threatening situation at the age of nineteen which resulted in a near-death experience. It occurred in Italy near the village of Fossalta during an artillery bombardment on July 18, 1918. An Austrian mortar shell landed very near the trench in which Hemingway had sought cover. The explosion caused several serious wounds and a loss of consciousness. His accompanying near-death experience was told to longtime journalist friend Guy Hickok of the *Brooklyn Daily Eagle:* "I felt my soul or something coming right out of my body like you'd pull a silk handkerchief out of a pocket by one corner. It flew around and then came back in and I wasn't dead anymore." This personal experience was later incorporated into *A Farewell to Arms* (Spraggett, 1974, pp. 72-73).

Louis Tucker, a Catholic priest, wrote a book published in 1943 entitled *Clerical Errors* wherein he describes his own near-death experience. The event took place in the spring of 1909 in Baton Rouge, Louisiana. Tucker was desperately ill from the effects of ptomaine poisoning. Consciousness began to slip away and he felt certain that he was about to die. The family physician arrived at the Tucker residence soon thereafter and subsequently pronounced him dead. What follows are the highlights of Tucker's experience.

The unconsciousness was short. The sensation was not quite like anything earthly; the nearest familiar thing to it is passing through a short tunnel on a train. There was the same sense of hurrying, of blackness, of rapid transition, of confused noise, and multiform, swift readjustment. Death is a very much overrated process. I have since suffered many times as much while waiting, under spinal block, for a comparatively minor surgical operation.

I emerged into a place where people were being met by friends. It was quiet and full of light, and Father was waiting for me. He looked exactly as he had in the last few years of his life and wore the last suit of clothes he had owned... I knew that the clothes Father wore were assumed because they were familiar to me, so that I might feel no strangeness in seeing him, and that to some lesser extent, his appearance was assumed also; I knew all these things by contagion, because he did.

...Soon I discovered that we were not talking, but thinking. I knew dozens of things that we did not mention because he knew them. He thought a question, I an answer, without speaking; the process was practically instantaneous. At the same time I caught his question I caught other things in his mind.... What he said was in ideas, no words: if I were to go back at all I must go at once... I did not want to go back; not in the least; the idea of self-preservation, the will to live was quite gone....

I swung into the blackness again, as a man might swing on a train, thoroughly disgusted that I could not stay, and absolutely certain that it was right for me to go back. That certainty has never wavered.

There was a short interval of confused and hurrying blackness and I came to, to find myself lying on my bed with the doctor bending over telling me that I was safe now and would live because circulation was re-established and my lips were no longer blue. I told him I knew that some time ago, and went to sleep. [Tucker, 1943, pp. 221-25]

Lord Geddes, a British professor and physician, presented an account of an individual who had "died" for a brief while and was later revived. He disclosed his patient's story before the members of the Royal Medical Society during their Edinburgh convention in 1937. The essential details were presented thus:

I suddenly realized that my consciousness was separating from another consciousness which was also me.... Gradually I realized that I could see not only my body and the bed in which it was, but everything in the whole house and garden, and then I realized that I was not only seeing things at home, but in London and in Scotland, in fact wherever my attention was directed...I was free in a time dimension of space, wherein "now" was in some way equivalent to "here"in the ordinary three dimensional space of everyday life. I next realized that my vision included not only "things" in the ordinary three dimensional places that I was in. Although I had no body, I had what appeared to be perfect two-eyed vision, and what I saw can only be described in this way, that I was conscious of a psychic stream flowing with life through time, and this gave me the impression of being visible, and it seemed to me to have a particularly intense iridescence. [Wheeler 1976, p. 56]

In his book, *Alone,* published in 1938, Admiral Richard Byrd discusses a near-death experience resulting from carbon monoxide poisoning during his famed Antarctica expedition.

Great waves of fear, a fear I had never known before, swept through me and settled deep within. But it wasn't the fear of suffering or even of death itself. It was the terrible anxiety over the consequences to those at home if I failed to return...Also during those hours of bitterness, I saw my whole life pass in review. I realized how wrong my sense of value had been and how I had failed to see that the simple, homely, unpretentious things of life are the most important....

The struggle went on interminably in a half-lighted borderland divided by a great white wall. Several times I was nearly across the wall into a field flooded with a golden light but each time I slipped back into a spinning darkness. Instinct plucked at my sleeve: You must wake up. You must wake up. I pinched the flesh over my ribs. I pulled my long hair. Then the tension eased; I fell across the wall; and instead of warm sunlight, I found myself in darkness, shivering from cold and thirsting for water. [Byrd 1938, pp. 118, 122]

In 1940, Irving Hallowell published an article in the *Journal of the Royal Anthropological Institute* entitled "Spirits of the Dead in Saulteaux Life and Thought." Hallowell spent several years in Canada studying the belief systems and observing the behavior of the aboriginal Berens River Saulteaux Indians. He detected a prevailing conviction in a life beyond death, a life regarded as beautiful and pleasant for all those making the "transition." Hallowell noted that this belief approached the order of direct knowledge and theorized that it was predicated much less on the basis of religious faith or superstitious illusion: "Aboriginal beliefs in the reality of a life beyond the grave cannot be viewed as simple dogmas that gain currency without any appeal to observation and experience (Hallowell, 1940, p. 29)."

Interestingly, Hallowell found that the convictions of the Berens River Saulteaux were a direct function of the testimony of individuals said to have passed through the curtain of death and returned to impart the fruits of their experience. He discovered that this "testimony" came from three different groups of individuals: (1) those who approached the land of the dead in a dream state; (2) those reputed to have been dead prior to successful resuscitation or resurrection; and (3) those who communicated with spirits of the dead in the "conjuring lodge." Persons who were believed to be dead or fatally ill were perceived as having visited the land of the dead within the context of direct firsthand experience. Their reflections carried relatively more weight among their fellow Saulteaux. Their reports, accordingly, constituted the primordial basis for Saulteaux convictions concerning life after death.

The "testimony" of these individuals revealed the following similarities in the near-death experience: (1) dissociation from the physical body occurred frequently; (2) there were often encounters with other entities in the "spirit realm," some of whom were thought to be loved ones and friends (significant others) who had previously died; and (3) death was depicted as blissful, peaceful, and pleasant— a happy event signifying the ultimate transition or passage to a better reality.

Another early near-death experience was reported by world-renowned psychologist Carl Gustav Jung in his autobiography, *Memories, Dreams, Reflections* (1961). The incident occurred early in 1944 when Jung suffered a heart attack. Jung, unconscious and receiving oxygen and camphor injections, recollects a profound altered state of consciousness. His experience involves a series of visionary impressions, mostly of the planet Earth, from a vantage point believed to be approximately a thousand miles high. He was presumably outside his physical body and enjoying the delights of markedly heightened perception.

I had the feeling that everything was being sloughed away; everything I had aimed at or wished for or thought, the whole phantasmagoria of earthly existence, fell away or was stripped from me—an extremely painful process. Nevertheless something remained; it was as if I now carried along with me everything I had ever experienced or done, everything that had happened around me. I might also say: it was with me, and I was it. I consisted of all that, so to speak. I consisted of my own history, and I felt with great certainty: this is what I am. I am this bundle of what has been and what has been accomplished...I would never have imagined that such experience was possible. It was not a product of imagination. The visions and experiences were utterly real; there was nothing subjective about them; they all had the quality of absolute objectivity....

I can describe the experience only as the ecstasy of a non-temporal state in which present, past, and future are one...."This is eternal bliss," I thought. "This cannot be described; it is far too wonderful. [Jung, p. 290]

In considering near-death experiences from an historical perspective, it is interesting to note that the man to whom Moody's best-selling book *Life After Life* (1975) is dedicated, psychiatrist George Ritchie, had his near-death experience in December of 1943, more than thirty years before *Life*'s publication. Ritchie's experience was among the first Moody came across and strongly influenced Moody's decision to research near-death phenomena. Consequently, one may infer that the very emergence of contemporary near-death research was inspired by and attributable to historical elements (to the degree that one perceives Moody's work as ground-breaking).

Another historical example of the near-death experience comes from the writings of Edward V. Rickenbacker. In his book *Rickenbacker: An Autobiography* he recorded the following observations of death as he felt it approaching:[5]

Then I began to die, I felt the presence of death, and I knew that I was going. Many people believe that dying is unpleasant, but that's not true. Dying is the sweetest, tenderest, most sensuous sensation. Death comes disguised as a sympathetic friend. All was serene and calm. How wonderful it would be simply to float out of this world. It is easy to die. You have to fight to live. [Wheeler, 1976, p. 36]

Curran (1975, p. 259) refers to a study of World War II military pilots who were involved in actual aircraft crashes. These subjects strongly felt that death was unavoidable during the incidents; they were each convinced that death would occur upon impact with the ground. Interestingly, Curran states that these pilots had amazingly astute memories of themselves during these episodes. Their sense of time was altered and what seemed like a long duration was actually only a few brief moments. Their experiences involved the flashback component wherein major if not all events of one's lifetime pass in review during the near-death episode.

Somerset Maugham, the British novelist, nearly died at the age of eighty in an English hospital. He was resuscitated after some members of the attending medical team believed him dead. Although Maugham was an avowed agnostic and a disbeliever in a life after death prior to the incident, his thinking changed radically following it. He described death as "a great final orgasm" and the ultimate in pleasurable experiences:

> Time ended; it might have been an hour or a century; the light began to change. To my surprise it did not grow darker but lighter; it became iridescent, blinding. I could sense my pulse fading and my heart beat slowing, and still the light increased in intensity, and then the most exquisite sense of release set in and continued, a great final spirit, a giving up of the whole being, body, spirit. All I knew was that the end had come and I remembered being grateful to nature for making it so exceedingly pleasant... Now that I know what death was like I need no longer be afraid of it. I can describe it accurately— natural death, I mean—I know nothing of violent death. Natural death is the final relaxation. Take it or leave it. [Kanin, 1973, p. 3]

During the 1950s, Dr. Robert Crookall, a British geologist, undertook a study of near-death experiences. He uncovered several cases where the out-of-the-body phenomenon was reported along with other elements of the Moody model. He observed that the out-of-the-body phenomenon reported in conjunction with near-death episodes was in many ways identical to reports from other persons who, although not involved in near-death episodes, had essentially the same kind of experience owing to other factors.[6] His work predates Moody and Kübler-Ross by more than two decades, yet his findings and observations are very similar to theirs (Crookall, 1961).

Ettinger (1964) discusses a near-death experience communicated by an elderly man who had been resuscitated. The man explained his impressions in this manner: "My pain was gone, and I couldn't feel my body. I heard the most peaceful music. The most beautiful music. God was there, and I was floating away. The music was all around me. I knew I was dead, but I wasn't afraid. Then the music stopped and you [the doctor] were leaning over me. It wasn't a dream" (Pandey, 1971, p. 5).

Battista (1964, pp. 83-84) comments that many of the physicians he has interviewed report that death is almost always preceded by "a perfect willingness to die." Despite the amount or intensity of previous suffering and pain among the dying patients attended by the physicians in his investigation, Battista found that the doctors noticed "an interval of perfect peace and often ecstasy before death" in almost all cases. He goes on to assert that there is no such thing as "death agony" except as it exists in the imagination. One pathologist in his sample of physicians observed that, on occasion, patients "may hear the ringing of nonexistent bells or see the flashing of nonexistent lights." (Many of the persons interviewed by Moody and other researchers have also discussed both these sensations.) He emphasized that his patients almost always died easily and painlessly.

Hunter (1967) published a case study of a thirty-four-year-old woman who reported a near-death experience stemming from an allergic reaction to penicillin. She reported witnessing, in rapid succession, various events from her childhood. She also recalled feelings of bliss and ecstasy as well as a vivid dream of the Taj Mahal. In a study of patients surviving cardiac arrest, Druss and Kornfeld (1967, p. 78) interviewed a total of ten resuscitees. One patient recalled nothing and therefore felt more assured that there is no life following death. Another stated that death is painless and that he no longer feared it because he had experienced it. A third reflected that "death does not involve a termination of perception, but rather, that some kind of perceiving goes on after life, as in a dream, that one continues to have visual images. All in all, the experience was not unpleasant." Thomas Hackett, as a physician on the staff of Massachusetts General Hospital in Boston, chanced upon yet another example of a pre-Moody, pre-Kübler-Ross near-death experience:

> Some time after the Apollo 14 moon shot I talked with a 57-year-old engineer who had just been resuscitated after arrest. He was quite elated at having survived that event and referred to it as "one of the most unique experiences of the 20th century, every bit as spectacular as landing on the moon." He spoke with pride of having crossed to the other side and returned none the worse. His attitude has persisted for nearly a year at this writing. [Hackett, 1972, pp. 136-37]

The historical accounts of near-death experiences presented in this section are further augmented by the work of Canning (1965),

MacMillan and Brown (1971), Noyes (1971), Noyes (1972), and Stevenson (1977). Most of these supplementary citations are discussed elsewhere in this volume.

CONCLUSIONS

The explicit aim of this paper has been to demonstrate a historical continuity and a compatible correlation between past and present accounts of near-death episodes and experiences. I have tried to reinforce the thesis that recoveries from deathlike states of being, and the epiphenomenal peak experiences which sometimes accompany them, span centuries of recorded human history and are decidedly not the exclusive product of our era. Improved medical technology and resuscitation techniques have only functioned to increase the frequency of such incidents (Moody, 1975, p. 100; 1977, pp. 103-4). It is important that this position be advanced by scholars and researchers of near-death phenomena if only to help dispel common myths and misconceptions in favor of a more comprehensive perspective.

It is not within the scope of this article to discuss theories and explanations surrounding near-death episodes and experiences. Different schools of thought have developed with different perspectives on the matter. There are those who assert that near-death experiences suggest a survival of bodily death. There are also those who have attempted to account for the phenomena within the framework of the physicalistic paradigm, that is, those who claim that near-death experiences are derivative of such things as cerebral anoxia, organic brain syndrome, depersonalization, or universal archetypes at the seat of consciousness. Regardless of the particular theoretical position one chooses, the element of historical linkages must necessarily enter into the equation. I hope this article has at least succeeded in lending further credence to the prominence and importance of this variable.

Notes

1. Although Elisabeth Kubler-Ross has not as yet formally published the findings of her near-death research, she has revealed the substance of her work through popular media (Kubler-Ross, 1975, 1976, 1977). I have learned in personal conversation with her that she has studied over one thousand cases of near-death experiences which bear an uncanny resemblance to those cases studied by Moody (1975, 1977).

2. The relationship between physiological and psychological precipitants of near-death experiences has definite implications in the search for causal explanations, since the imagery reported by both groups of individuals has compelling similarity. There are data, albeit a small quantity, which indicate that the same motifs are present in both samples. This may suggest that the phenomena of near-death experiences has a necessary connection to one or the other conditions, but presumably not to both in any concomitant combination.

3. Further discussion of Heim's work along with other historical examples of near-death experiences, can be found in Grof and Halifax (1978, pp. 131-57). Their presentation of this material is truly excellent and most informative.

4. Beaufort's story was printed in the London Daily News on January 15, 1858 and was published again in a book entitled *Euthanasia or Medical Treatment in Aid of an Easy Death* by W. Munk (New York: Longmans, Green, 1887).

5. These impressions of death came to Rickenbacker shortly before his own life ended. Many persons, just before the moment of their actual death, have described visions which are sometimes analogous to those appearing in accounts of near-death experiences. See *At the Hour of Death* by Karlis Osis, and Erlendur Haraldsson (New York: Avon Books, 1977).

6. The out-of-the-body aspect of the near-death experience has been referred to by Sabom and Kreutziger (1977, p. 649) as "autoscopy" or "self-visualization from a detached position of height." Others have dubbed it "astral projection." Regardless of the label one chooses to apply, it is referred to as an altered state of consciousness where perception and locomotion take place ostensibly outside of and independent of the physical body and its sensory mechanisms. Parapsychologists and others have argued that the near-death episode is not the exclusive precipitant of out-of-the-body states; that such states can occur for other reasons such as fasting, meditation, or psychedelic drug ingestion. Crookall was perhaps the first individual to call attention to this relationship.

References

Battista, O.A. 1964. "What Happens When You Die." *Science Digest* 55:5, 80-84.

Becker, Ernest. 1973. *The Denial of Death*. New York: Free Press.

Byrd, Richard A. 1938. *Alone*. New York: Ace Books.

Canning, Raymond R. 1965. "Mormon Return-from-the-Dead Stories: Fact or Folklore." *Utah Academy Proceedings* 42:29-37. (Summarized in *Sociology of Death* by Glenn M. Vernon, New York: Ronald Press, 1970.)

Crookall, Robert. 1961. *The Supreme Adventure.* London: James Clarke.

Curran, Charles A. 1975. "Death and Dying." *Journal of Religion and Health* 4:254-64.

Dlin, Barney M., Andrew Stern, and Steven J. Poliakoff. 1974. "Survivors of Cardiac Arrest: The First Few Days." *Psychosomatics* 15:61-67.

Druss, Richard G., and Donald S. Kornfeld. 1967. "The Survivors of Cardiac Arrest: A Psychiatric Study." *JAMA* 201:75-80.

Ettinger, Robert. 1964. *The Prospect of Immortality.* New York: Doubleday.

Garfield, Charles A. 1979. Summary of findings from a recent investigation of persons near death. *Anabiosis* 1:3-6.

Greyson, Bruce, and Ian Stevenson. 1978. "Research Brief: A Phenomenological Analysis of Near-Death Experiences." Paper presented at the 21st Annual Convention of the Parapsychological Association, August 8-12, 1978, Washington University, St. Louis, Mo.

Grof, Stanislav, and Joan Halifax. 1977. *The Human Encounter with Death.* New York: Dutton.

Hackett, Thomas P. 1972. "The Lazarus Complex Revisited." *Annals of Internal Medicine* 76:135-37.

Hallowell, Irving. 1940. "Spirits of the Dead in Saulteaux Life and Thought." *Journal of the Royal Anthropological Institute* 70:29-51.

Heim, Albert. 1972. "Remarks on Fatal Falls." *Yearbook of the Swiss Alpine Club* (1892) 27:327-37. (Trans. by Russell Noyes and Roy Kletti, *Omega* 3:45-52.)

Hunter, R.C.A. 1967. "On the Experience of Nearly Dying." *American Journal of Psychiatry* 124:122-26.

Jung, Carl. 1961. *Memories, Dreams, Reflections.* New York: Pantheon.

Kaempffert, Waldemar. 1953. "What Is Clinical Death?" *Science Digest* 34:2.

Kanin, Garson. 1973. *Remembering Mr. Maugham.* New York: Bantam Books.

Kastenbaum, Robert, and Ruth Aisenberg. 1976. *The Psychology of Death.* New York: Springer Pub. Co.

Kübler-Ross, Elisabeth. 1975. "Life After Death: Yes, Beyond a Shadow of a Doubt." Interview in an article by Linda Witt, *People* 4:21, 66-69.

————. 1976. "There Is Life After Death." Interview in an article by Kenneth L. Woodward, *McCall's,* August 1976, pp. 97-139; see also "Life After Death?" by Kenneth L. Woodward, *Newsweek,* July 12, 1976, p. 41.

————. 1977. "The Miracle of Kübler-Ross." Interview in an article by Ann Nietzke, *Human Behavior* 6:9, 18-27.

Langone, John. 1972. *Death Is a Noun: A View of the End of Life.* New York: Dell.

MacMillan, R.L., and K.W.G. Brown. 1971. "Cardiac Arrest Remembered." *Canadian Medical Association Journal* 104:889-90.

Mant, A. Keith. 1976. "The Medical Definition of Death." In *Death: Current Perspectives,* ed. by Edwin S. Shneidman. Palo Alto, Cal.: Mayfield Pub. Co.

Moody, Raymond A. 1975. *Life After Life.* New York: Bantam Books.

————. 1977. *Reflections on Life After Life.* New York: Bantam Books.

Negovskii, V.A. 1962. *Resuscitation and Artificial Hypothermia.* New York: Consultants Bureau.

Noyes, Russell, 1971. "Dying and Mystical Consciousness." *Journal of Thanatology* 1:25-41.

Noyes, Russell. 1972. "The Experience of Dying," *Psychiatry* 35:174-84.

Noyes, Russell, and Roy Kletti. 1976. "Depersonalization in the Face of Life-Threatening Danger: A Description." *Psychiatry* 39:19-27.

Pandey, Carol. 1971. "The Need for the Psychological Study of Clinical Death." *Omega* 2:1-9.

Pfister, Otto. 1930. "Shockdenken und shockphantasien bei hochster todesgefahr." *Zeitschrift fuer Psychoanalytische Padagogik* 16: 430-55.

Rawlings, Maurice. 1978. *Beyond Death's Door.* Nashville: Nelson Pub. Co.

Ring, Ken. 1978. "Some Determinants of the Prototypic Near-Death Experience." Paper presented at the Twenty-First Annual Convention of the Parapsychological Association, August 8-12, 1978, Washington University, St. Louis, Mo.

Rogo, D. Scott. 1979. "Research on Deathbed Experiences: Some Contemporary and Historical Perspectives." *Journal of the Academy of Religion and Psychical Research* 2:37-49.

Sabom, Michael and Sarah Kreutziger. 1977. "Near-Death Experiences." *Florida Medical Journal* 64:648-50.

Spraggett, Allen. 1974. *The Case for Immortality.* New York: New American Library.

Stevenson, Ian. 1977. "Research into the Evidence of Man's Survival After Death: A Historical and Critical Survey with a Summary of Recent Developments." *Journal of Nervous and Mental Disease* 165:152-70.

Tart, Charles C. 1972. "States of Consciousness and State Specific Sciences." *Science:* 176:1203-10.

Tucker, Louis. 1943. *Clerical Errors.* New York: Harper and Brothers.

Wheeler, David R. 1976. *Journey to the Other Side.* New York: Tempo Books.

PART THREE

Recent Research on
Near-Death Experiences

3

Cardiac Arrest Remembered

R.L. MacMillan and K.W.G. Brown

A SIXTY-EIGHT-YEAR-OLD MAN WHO previously had suffered no symptoms of coronary artery disease awoke with aching pain in the left arm. Squeezing retrosternal pain developed several hours later and persisted until his admission to hospital in the late afternoon. He was transferred without delay to the coronary unit, where his general condition was found to be satisfactory. Blood pressure was 126/78, heart sounds were normal and there were no signs of cardiac failure. A 12-lead electrocardiogram was normal. The heart rhythm was monitored continuously and only an occasional ventricular premature beat was seen that followed the T wave by a comfortable distance. Ten hours after admission the chest pain became worse and the patient was given 50 mg. of meperidine. Suddenly a ventricular premature beat fell on a T wave, causing ventricular fibrillation. One of the coronary unit nurses recognized the cardiac arrest and immediately defibrillated the patient. After this there were no further serious arrhythmias, and convalescence was uneventful apart from an episode of pulmonary infarction. The ECG was normal the morning after defibrillation, and it was not until the 10th day that changes of anterior subendocardial infarction became evident. Changes in SGOT and CPK levels, however,

Cardiac Arrest Remembered" by R.L. MacMillan and K.W.G. Brown, *Canadian Medical Association Journal*, 104 (May 22, 1971):889-90. Copyright © 1971 by Canadian Medical Association. Reprinted by permission of the publisher and the authors.

were diagnostic of recent myocardial infarction from the first day in hospital. The patient remembered in detail the events surrounding his cardiac arrest, and the following account is his own vivid description of his experience. (The right leg mentioned was badly scarred from osteomyelitis suffered in childhood.)

As I promised, I am setting down my experiences as I remember them when I had the cardiac arrest last May.

I find it hard to describe certain parts—I do not have words to express how vivid the experience was. The main thing that stands out is the clarity of my thoughts during the episode. They were almost exactly as I have written them and in retrospect it seems that they are fixed in my memory—more so than other things that have happened to me. It seemed at times that I was having a "dual" sensation— actually experiencing certain things yet at the same time "seeing" myself during these experiences.

I had been admitted into the Intensive Care ward in the early evening. I remember looking at my wrist watch and it appeared to be a few minutes before 4 a.m. I was lying flat on my back because of the intravenous tubes and the wires to the recording machine. Just then I gave a very, very deep sigh and my head flopped over to the right. I thought "Why did my head flop over?—I didn't move it—I must be going to sleep." This was apparently my last conscious thought.

Then I am looking at my own body from the waist up, face to face (as though through a mirror in which I appear to be in the lower left corner). Almost immediately I saw myself leave my body, coming out through my head and shoulders (I did not see my lower limbs). The "body" leaving me was not exactly in vapour form, yet it seemed to expand very slightly once it was clear of me. It was somewhat transparent, for I could see my other "body" through it. Watching this I thought "So this is what happens when you die" (although no thought of being dead presented itself to me).

Suddenly I am sitting on a very small object travelling at great speed, out and up into a dull blue-grey sky, at a 45-degree angle. I thought "It's lonely out here.—Where am I going to end up?—This is one journey I must take alone."

Down below to my left I saw a pure white cloud-like substance also moving up on a line that would intersect my course. Somehow I was able to go down and take a look at it. It was perfectly rectangular in shape (about the same proportions as a regular building brick), but full of holes (like a sponge). Two thoughts came to me: "What will happen to me when it engulfs me?" and "You don't have to worry; it

has all happened before and everything will be taken care of." I have
no recollection of the shape catching up with me.

My next sensation was of floating in a bright, pale yellow light—a
very delightful feeling. Although I was not conscious of having any
lower limbs, I felt something being torn off the scars of my right leg,
as if a large piece of adhesive tape had been taken off. I thought
"They have always said your body is made whole out here. I wonder
if my scars are gone," but though I tried I could not seem to locate my
legs. I continued to float, enjoying the most beautiful tranquil
sensation. I had never experienced such a delightful sensation and
have no words to describe it.

Then there were sledge-hammer blows to my left side. They
created no actual pain, but jarred me so much that I had difficulty in
retaining my balance (on whatever I was sitting). After a number of
these blows, I began to count them and when I got to six I said (aloud
I think), "What the...are you doing to me?" and opened my eyes.

Immediately I was in control of all my faculties and recognized the
doctors and nurses around me. I asked the head nurse at the foot of
my bed, "What's happening?" and she replied that I'd had a bad turn.
I then asked who had been kicking me, and a doctor pointed to a
nurse on my left, remarking that she really had to "thump" me hard
and that I would be black and blue on my left side the next day (I
don't think I was).

Just a few comments as I think over what happened to me. I
wonder if the bright yellow surroundings could have been caused by
someone looking into my eyes with a bright light?

I have read about heart transplants where it is claimed the brain
dies before the heart stops. In my case, my brain must have been
working after my heart stopped beating for me to experience these
sensations.

If death comes to a heart patient in this manner, no one has cause
to worry about it. I felt no pain (other than what I had when I entered
hospital), and while it was a peculiar experience it was not
unpleasant. The floating part of my sensation was so strangely
beautiful that I said to a doctor later that night, "If I go out again,
don't bring me back—it's so beautiful out there," and at that time I
meant it.

It is unusual for patients to remember the events surrounding
cardiac arrest. More often there is a period of amnesia of several
hours' duration before and after the event. This description is
extremely interesting. The patient saw himself leaving his body and

was able to observe it "face to face". This could be the concept of the soul leaving the body which is found in many religions. The delightful feeling of floating in space and the tranquility, the yellow light, the rectangular shape with holes in it, associated with the wish of not wanting to be brought back again, may provide comfort and reassurance to patients suffering from coronary artery disease as well as to their relatives.

4

Depersonalization in the Face of Life-Threatening Danger: A Description

Russell Noyes, Jr., and Roy Kletti

PERSONS SUDDENLY THREATENED WITH death have often reported a variety of mental phenomena as part of a progressive deviation from normal consciousness. These have been described by people rescued at the last moment from drownings, falls, and similar accidents. Some anecdotal reports of subjective experiences during mortal danger exist in autobiographical as well as clinical sources (Noyes 1972). However, the first study of them was undertaken in 1892 by Albert Heim, who accumulated the accounts of over 30 survivors of falls in the Alps. He claimed that in nearly every instance a similar mental state developed, which he characterized dramatically as follows:

> There was no anxiety, no trace of despair, no pain; but rather calm seriousness, profound acceptance, and a dominant mental quickness and sense of surety. Mental activity became enormous, rising to a hundred-fold velocity or intensity. The relationships of events and their probable outcomes were overviewed with objective clarity. No confusion entered at all. Time became greatly expanded. . . . In many

cases there followed a sudden review of the individual's entire past; and finally the person falling often heard beautiful music and fell in a superbly blue heaven containing roseate cloudlets. [Noyes and Kletti, 1972, pp. 46-47]

What follows is a descriptive analysis of 114 accounts of near-death experiences obtained from 104 persons.

The accounts of the experiences were collected in several ways: 16 persons were personally interviewed when it was learned that they had survived extreme danger; another 38 responded to mountaineering journal advertisements for accounts of subjective experiences during dangerous falls; 39 offered unsolicited reports of their experiences in response to news items regarding this inquiry; and finally, 11 accounts were obtained through a variety of personal contacts. Each person was encouraged to submit a detailed account of his experience and complete a brief questionnaire.

The questionnaire was completed by 85 persons. It contained 40 questions calling for "yes" or "no" answers. The first four dealt with factors presumed to influence the experience. The first asked each person whether or not he believed he had been about to die during his accident. Three more questions dealt with the meaning attached to the experience. The remainder inquired about a variety of subjective phenomena commonly reported during depersonalization and mystical states of consciousness.

The life-threatening circumstances responsible for the experiences reported were as follows: falls, 47; drownings, 16; automobile accidents, 14; serious illnesses, 10; battlefield explosions, 6; cardiac arrests, 5; allergic reactions, 4; and miscellaneous accidents, 12. Accounts were obtained from 70 men and 34 women having a mean age of 33 years. The average (median) age of respondents at the time of their experience was 24 years. The data presented in this article were gathered informally and those who offered their experiences may have been prompted to do so by curiosity about them. In spite of this bias, the accounts are of great interest and, in view of their numbers, warrant serious consideration.

FINDINGS

The frequency with which various subjective phenomena were reported during moments of extreme danger is shown in the table. Persons who had believed that they were about to die (column 1) experienced them more frequently than those who had not thought

Subjective Phenomena During Extreme Danger

*Percentage of Subjects**

Subjective Phenomena	Death Believed Imminent (*N* = 59)	Death Not Believed Imminent (*N* = 26)	Total (*N* = 85)
Altered passage of time	80%	65%	75
Unusually vivid thoughts	71	62	68
Increased speed of thoughts	69	68	68
Sense of detachment	67	56	64
Feeling of unreality	67	54	63
Automatic movements	64	52	60
Lack of emotion	54	46	50
Detachment from body	54	38	49
Sharper vision or hearing	49	38	46
Revival of memories	47	12	36
Great understanding	43	24	37
Colors or visions	41	24	36
Sense of harmony or unity	39	24	35
Control by external force	37	25	32
Objects small or far away	36	33	35
Vivid mental images	36	12	29
Voices, music, or sounds	25	14	23

*Based on those completing questionnaire.

themselves close to death (column 2). A number of distinct elements were particularly characteristic of the experience, and following a presentation of examples, will be described in detail. These include altered perception of time, lack of emotion, feeling of unreality, altered attention, sense of detachment, loss of control, revival of memories, and ineffability.

Example 1

A 24-year-old stock car driver experienced two potentially fatal racing accidents in a single year. The first happened on a straight-away as he was traveling over a hundred miles an hour. In the course of the accident his car was thrown 30 feet in the air and turned over several times before landing on its wheels. He said:

> As soon as I saw him I knew I was going to hit him. I remember thinking that death or injury was coming but after that I didn't feel much at all. It seemed like the whole thing took forever. Everything was in slow motion and it seemed to me like I was a player on a stage and could see myself tumbling over and over in the car. It was as though I sat in the stands and saw it all happening. I realized I was

definitely in danger but I was not frightened. While I was up in the air I felt like I was floating.... I saw flashes of color and distinctly remember blues, greens, and yellows. Everything was so strange....

As soon as I left the ground, I seemed to leave reality and move into another world. At that point I noticed how much sharper my vision was. I could see things more clearly and distinctly than at any time in my life. I remember being upside down and, looking backwards, I saw the man who won the race pass under me. That guy was looking up and I can still see the amazed look on his face. The whole experience was like a dream but at no time did I lose my sense of where I was.... It was like floating on air.... Finally, the car pancaked itself on the track and I was jolted back to reality.

This account illustrates the slowing of time, lack of emotion, sense of unreality, feeling of detachment, and heightening of certain perceptions, coupled with a dulling of others. The author's use of metaphors to describe his experience is noteworthy; his description has an "as if" quality throughout.

Example 2

A 21-year-old college senior described her reaction when, as a result of swerving to miss an oncoming automobile, she lost control of her car. Seeing a bridge abutment looming ahead, she knew she was about to die. And at that point:

...despite the horror of the situation, I entered a calm dreamlike state accompanied by a feeling of being at peace with everything. Then I saw an endless stream of past experiences—there must have been hundreds—go through my mind. All sound seemed to blur into an indescribable monotone and all of this became superimposed upon the scene actually taking place. I cannot remember specific thoughts or experiences that passed through my mind, but there were many and they were all pleasant. During all of this, time stood still. It seemed to take forever for everything to happen. Space too was unreal. It was all very much like sitting in a movie theater and watching it happen on the screen. I didn't feel like a participant much of the time....

This young woman gives a typical description of the altered perception of time and space, lack of emotion, and sense of detachment. The redirection of her attention toward memories of past experiences that blotted out environmental perceptions is also noteworthy.

Example 3

A 24-year-old mountain climber described the mental events which accompanied two falls, either one of which might have resulted in his death. Having lost his footing during a descent, he attempted a self-arrest but lost his ice axe in the process. Finding himself helplessly exposed to a 2,000-foot drop, he reported:

> I seemed to lose hope of saving myself but somehow reacted with an instinct for survival, grabbing whatever I could with my hands. Perhaps my subconscious mind initiated this reaction because consciously I was aware of negative thoughts. Losing my ice axe seemed to put control of the situation in the hands of God.... I felt intense fear; my thoughts speeded up; time slowed down; and my attention was redirected toward survival and deeply imbedded memories.... My mind seemed to alternate between perceiving and thinking. While perceptions were being registered, my thinking seemed to stop; and, while thinking, my data-gathering processes were at work, but perceptions were not registered in my memory. I saw and heard the events of my fall in vivid detail.... Some of my thoughts were of future events, I pictured my companion and myself falling 2,000 feet to our deaths. I thought of my mother and what she would think if I were dead. Other thoughts included spiritual perceptions. I felt closer to God. I developed an understanding of death as something beautiful, a realization that stands out yet today as profoundly important. At times my thoughts were so intense that my senses seemed numb. Memories of earlier dangerous experiences were revived but were not vivid.

This account illustrates the heightening, narrowing, and redirecting of attention that were characteristic of the experiences reported. A revival of memories and phenomena having religious significance are briefly mentioned.

Example 4

Religious significance also appeared in the account of a 14-year-old boy who accidentally shot himself in the chest. The religious content was enriched by visions that he recognized as unreal at the time. He said that as soon as he shot himself:

> I became aware of a burning pain in my stomach and a deafening ringing in my ears, but the thing I noticed especially was the odor of gun smoke, which was painfully strong. Everywhere I looked I saw a deep blue color. I found myself lying on the floor and I believed I was

going to die. My father rushed in then and urged me to get up, but he didn't seem to be speaking to me at all. Then the room filled with people that weren't actually there, including my girlfriend, a cousin, and my grandmother. They all appeared as they normally would, but none seemed to notice me. When I got up and walked out (I fell once before reaching the car), it seemed to me that strength came from a force outside myself. It affected my mind as well as my body, and I think it enabled me to hold onto life.

When I reached the car, my attention became riveted on memories of my early life. They began when I was about three and continued up to the present. I saw myself in a high chair at age three. I was with my father under a bridge when we caught a prize paddlefish. I saw myself with friends. The memories were pleasant but made me sad, realizing that this was the life I was leaving. They were very clear, almost as though I were actually living them. Many were events I had not recalled before. They must have been moving extremely rapidly although they did not seem to at the time. My thoughts were speeded up and time seemed stretched out. I felt numb and detached from what was going on around me.... In the emergency room I found myself outside of my body, as though I were standing off to one side. I saw myself as plainly as if I had been there; I appeared to be in pain.

This dramatic account provides an illustration of each of the elements listed above. The youth's descriptions of early memories (panoramic memory) and of detachment from his body are particularly vivid.

Example 5

A mystical extension of the phenomena so far described may be found in the following account. A 22-year-old woman, in a serious suicide attempt, took an overdose of barbiturates. The alteration in consciousness produced by the drug no doubt influenced the development of the mystical experience, in addition to her awareness of impending death. Not long after taking the overdose she began to feel drowsy and then:

...as I went deeper, reality vanished and visions, soft lights, and an extreme feeling of calm acceptance passed over me like waves. The waves seemed to massage a part of me, but not my physical body. I saw lovely things and took leave of the phases of my life. I said goodby to myself as I watched the various stages. I felt close enough to grab onto some sort of wheel which I would become one with, yet add to. I would be filled with the wisdom of things I'd wondered about but would be myself no longer. I would diffuse, burst apart. I felt close to knowing all and accepting a long rest and lasting peace. My experiences were close to being in no time at all, almost as though time were at a standstill. Things were very far away, almost in another world. I couldn't touch them. My strength was centered but scattered. I was stronger because of being more whole, because I was no longer me as I had once known myself. I had a feeling of becoming part of a greater whole, a feeling impossible for me to describe exactly. It was a loss of identity, and not a feeling I could relate to the realm of human experience.

In this account many of the components—such as alteration in time and space, detachment, and recall of early experiences—are recognizable but in extreme, symbolic, or ineffable form.

CHARACTERISTIC ELEMENTS

The most frequently reported subjective phenomenon experienced during extreme danger was an apparent slowing of time (75%; see table). This was outer or environmental time, as opposed to inner time, which was perceived as being correspondingly increased in speed. Not only did elapsed time seem drawn out, but events seemed to happen in slow motion. Yet in contrast to the outward slowing, individuals described their thoughts as speeded up (68%) and expressed amazement at the number of thoughts or mental images that passed through their minds in a matter of seconds. These two aspects of the experience of time were generally described together and were clearly related to one another.

Lack of emotion was a striking feature of the experience for 50% of those completing the questionnaires. Many experienced fear momentarily upon the recognition of extreme danger. However, they soon found themselves calm. Nearly half reported no fear at all despite the gravity of the situation. A third acknowledged feeling as though a wall existed between themselves and their feelings. Emotions were not entirely blocked out, however, for 52% reported fear; 37%, sadness; and 30%, anger. Rarely painful, these emotions were dampened and, when recognized at all, were of minimal intensity. Under the circumstances described, most respondents found themselves calm and peaceful. In fact, many described their emotional state as pleasurable and 23% even experienced joy. A 67-year-old physician, recalling his narrow escape from drowning 50 years earlier, said, "... once I realized I could not rescue myself, an indescribable feeling of calmness and serenity came over me that I have often wished desperately to experience again." And a 30-year-old mountaineer who lost his footing in a creek that was plunging down the side of a mountain claimed that, having resigned himself to his fate, "I had no more feeling of anxiety. In fact, at that moment I became elated." As in both of these instances, pleasurable emotions generally appeared when the person gave in to his presumed fate. Anger, on the other hand, was more commonly reported by persons who persisted in rescue efforts throughout the period of danger.

More than half (63%) of those completing questionnaires indicated that they had felt strange or unreal during their experience; 31% felt as though the world about them were unreal; a smaller number reported feeling as though the accident were not actually happening to them. Despite this sense of separation from reality, an appreciation of it was maintained throughout. This fact was clear from the metaphorical language used in describing experiences and repeated use of the phrases "as if" and "as though." A landing craft commander who was nearly killed when an enemy ammunition stockpile blew up beside him felt "as if I were sitting on a cloud looking down upon the whole scene, past, present, and future. Tremendous explosions were occurring all around me but faded and because a minor part of the whole experience." Thus, while removed from reality, he nevertheless maintained his contact with it.

Attention appeared to be heightened and narrowly focused. During a fall which he expected to be fatal, a 19-year-old mountain climber reported:

> Not only were my thought processes speeded up, but I was aware of a definite and intense deviation from normal consciousness. The intense fear and subconscious hope of survival instinctively forced a concentration of my thoughts on rescue efforts and a redirection of my whole mind onto whatever might be necessary to prevent the potential plunge. For example, if I had been cold, I would not have felt it. If I had been hurting myself, I would have felt no pain.... My vision was very active and alert.

Thus, within the immediate focus of attention, whether on perceptions or mental images, objects became increasingly vivid, whereas outside this focus perceptions and sensations were dulled or obscured entirely. So long as an individual persisted in efforts to rescue himself, this vastly increased alertness was directed, as necessary, toward accomplishing this end. A jet pilot during the Vietnam conflict claimed that this altered state of mind saved him from almost certain death when his plane was improperly launched. He said:

> ...when the nose-wheel strut collapsed I vividly recalled, in a matter of about three seconds, over a dozen actions necessary to successful recovery of flight attitude. The procedures I needed were readily available. I had almost total recall and felt in complete control. I seemed to be doing everything that I could and doing it properly.

Many persons felt, as in the case of this jet pilot, that they performed feats, both mental and physical, of which they would ordinarily have been incapable. However, once such efforts were given up, attention seemed to turn inward, leading to further reflection upon unalterable circumstances and life's approaching end.

A sense of detachment was reported by a majority of persons surviving these moments of extreme danger (64%). One mountain climber noted that although his fall of 30 feet had not taken long, he found "ample time in a peculiarly calm and impersonal way" to think that he would probably die. "It is difficult," he commented, "to describe the odd third-person viewpoint I seemed to have during the fall." Many spoke of feeling like observers rather than participants in the events taking place. Half (49%) claimed to have experienced a feeling of being detached from their bodies. Occasionally this detached, "observing" self was described as traveling outside of space and time.

A majority of subjects (60%) reported a sense of loss of control, consisting of feeling as though movements or thoughts were mechanical or automatic. A more exaggerated sense of loss of control took the form of feeling in the presence or under the control of an outside force (32%). A young woman claimed that when she had been on the verge of death following a serious automobile accident that occurred as she was on her way to her honeymoon, she "felt the presence of someone or something with the power of life and death within me.... I talked to the being and said that my life had been so gratifying that if it were my time to go, it was acceptable to me."

A dramatic accompaniment of many near-death experiences was a revival of memories (36%). This occurred largely among persons expecting to die (see table, p. 53) and commonly took a form called panoramic memory. Scenes of early life passed through the person's mind rapidly "as though on a conveyer belt" or "like a film sprung loose from the camera," suggesting a loss in the continuity of images, one from the next. The scenes depicted were vivid and were often accompanied by emotions appropriate to their content. All were memories of presumed actual events, some of which had not previously been recalled. Most were pleasurable, although painful remembrances were also reported. One young woman who had suddenly been confronted with the probability that complications of a serious automobile accident would be fatal said:

> ...my life passed before me in a way that took me right back to my childhood. I remembered the smell of pudding my mother used to make, the smell of the old house, and feelings I had then. These were things long forgotten. The memories were beautiful and I was happy to have experienced them.

Very early memories were reported as often as later ones, and they frequently appeared in sequence.

The ineffable quality of these reactions to moments of extreme danger was repeatedly commented upon: 38% found their experiences hard to describe. Many found language inadequate to communicate experiences that were so foreign. Their difficulty was often compounded by a reluctance to speak of events that might reflect on their sanity or, because of their mystical nature, might invite criticism. However, great personal significance was often attached to these experiences, an aspect discussed elsewhere (Noyes and Kletti, in press).

Mystical consciousness, as it is commonly defined (James 1929; Stace 1960), appeared to be an extension or further elaboration of the deviation of consciousness thus far described. It seemed not so much a distinct element of the altered mental state under examination but rather its most extreme progression. Characteristic components of this mystical extension included transcendence of time and space, feelings of unity, loss of will, sense of truth, and intense emotion. For someone who had progressed to this point, not only was the perception of time altered but also the person often perceived of himself as outside of or beyond time, so that his experience took on a timeless quality. Similarly, space often appeared limitless. Not only did his movements seem automatic, but he frequently felt as though his "will were in abeyance, and indeed sometimes as if he were grasped and held by a superior power" (James 1929, pp. 380-81). And, finally, separated from his body and freed from the limits of his being, he often became united with the universe.

The following brief account is illustrative of this transcendence of time, space, and individual identity. A 55-year-old man recalled his experience as a soldier during World War II when his jeep was blown up by a German mine. He reported:

> Almost immediately after the explosion, I was certain that death had occurred. I experienced no physical sensations, no sense perceptions. Rather I seemed to have entered a state in which only my thoughts or mind existed. I felt total serenity and peace. I had no remembrance of anything, only a realization that life had ended and that my mind was continuing to exist. I had no realization of time passing, only of one moment which never altered. Neither did I have any concept of space, since my existence seemed only mental. I cannot stress strongly enough the feeling of total peace of mind and of total blissful acceptance of my new status, which I knew would be never-ending.

The sense of truth characteristic of this mystical extension of consciousness suggests that an increasing separation from familiar reality develops as the observing self is progressively engulfed by the experience.

A sense of harmony or unity was reported by a third of the subjects who completed questionnaires (35%). Similarly, a third reported a feeling of great understanding (37%). It is noteworthy that the mystical extension of this experience occurred almost exclusively in persons in whom some alteration in cerebral functioning might be presumed to have occurred, judging from the circumstances of their experiences. Such an alteration might be assumed, for example, in the case of drownings or serious illnesses but not in the case of falls or automobile accidents uncomplicated by head injuries.

DISCUSSION

The subjective phenomena herein described in reaction to mortal danger are, for the most part, the same ones identified by Slater and Roth (1969, pp. 119-24) in their excellent review of depersonalization. The syndrome, especially as it occurs in patients, has been described by a number of authors (Ackner 1954; Mayer-Gross

1935). A classic early description was provided by Schilder in 1928 (p. 32):

> To the depersonalized individual the world appears strange, peculiar, foreign, dreamlike. Objects appear at times strangely diminished in size, at times flat. Sounds appear to come from a distance. The tactile characteristics of objects likewise seem strangely altered. But the patients complain not only of the changes in their perceptivity but their imagery appears to be altered. The patients characterize their imagery as pale, colorless, and some complain that they have altogether lost the power of imagination. The emotions likewise undergo marked alterations. The patients complain that they are capable of experiencing neither pain nor pleasure, love and hate have perished within them. They experience a fundamental change in their personality, and the climax is reached with their complaints that they have become strangers to themselves. It is as though they were dead, lifeless, mere automatons.

The syndrome accompanies a variety of mental disorders and altered states of consciousness. It frequently occurs in normal people as well, but since the majority of observations have been made on patients, differences in the phenomena observed in the presumably normal population reported on here are worth examining. It is safe to assume that the syndrome developed as a normal reaction to suddenly-presented, life-threatening danger. It seems clearly to have represented an adaptive, even life-saving, response in many instances. At what point the response may have become disorganized and what phenomena may represent such a breakdown is difficult to determine.

The chief difference observed in persons exposed to extreme danger was an alteration in attention. Depersonalized patients have not reported a heightening of perception but have, instead, rather consistently complained of a generalized dulling or numbing of perception and mental imagery. Likewise, a speeding of mental processes has not been typical of patient reports. While environmental events have seemed to progress slowly for them, they have not described a corresponding acceleration of mental processes. During extreme danger the focus of attention appears to become sharply narrowed. Within a restricted focus, mental images are intensified, even to the extreme of appearing as perceptions. And some sensations and perceptions normally on the periphery of the sphere of immediate attention are excluded from awareness entirely.

A very similar alteration in attention occurs in marijuana intoxication, a comparison specifically referred to by several persons in their accounts. James (1890) likened this change in attention to the effect of observing events taking place through a microscope. Passing at their normal rate, events seen through the high-powered lens would be seen vividly but would appear to flow more rapidly, would take on a two-dimensional quality, and would, at the same time, appear to lose their context within a larger field.

A revival of memories is yet another feature not found among patients suffering from depersonalization. However, as will be explained elsewhere, this particular component appears to be more closely related to life-threatening circumstances than to depersonalization per se (Noyes and Kletti, in press). On the other hand, the vivid, two-dimensional, high-speed qualities of the memories are probably determined by that syndrome. Certainly their occurrence is no myth, though their frequency remains undetermined.

In contrast to Ackner's (1954) characterization of patients as distressed by the emotional blunting they experience, persons confronted with sudden threats to their lives were gratified at finding themselves calm in the face of the most frightening circumstances imaginable. In fact, many remarked that dying in such a manner would scarcely be distressing. Beyond that, the reaction pattern, by attenuating fear, prevented the paralyzing or disorganizing panic that might so easily have developed in such moments. And, attesting to the effectiveness of this mechanism, many commented that they had been without frightening dreams or anxiety after their accidents and also that they had not found memory of the accident disturbing.

Mystical phenomena, according to James (1929), are transient. They have been reported as a part of brief depersonalization experiences of young people but, not surprisingly, have been absent from the chronically depersonalized states of patients. Naturally occurring mystical states of consciousness commonly develop during periods of intense emotional arousal and alterations in conciousness of various types. Both conditions were frequently present under the circumstances described.

CONCLUSION

From our examination of near-death experiences we may conclude that what Heim (1892) wrote over eighty years ago was substantially correct. He described a syndrome commonly reported by emotionally disturbed patients to which the term depersonalization was later applied. The differences between the subjective experiences of individuals in the midst of life-threatening danger and depersonalization developing among patients may add to our understanding of this curious disorder. Heim intended his presentation as a consolation to the families of victims of mountain-climbing accidents. Similarly, one may today take comfort from the fact that, suddenly confronted by death, he might find within himself the resources for coping with that frightful prospect. In such an urgent moment, strength might be found to effect a rescue, but failing in that, to face life's end with serenity, even acceptance.

References

Ackner, B. 1954. "Depersonalization. I. Aetiology and Phenomenology." *J. Mental Sci.* 100:838-53.

Heim, A. 1892. "Remarks on Fatal Falls." *Yearbook of the Swiss Alpine Club* 27:327-37; trans. by R. Noyes and R. Kletti, 1972, *Omega* 3:45-52.

James, W. 1890. *Principles of Psychology.* Vol. 1. New York: MacMillan.

James, W. 1929. *The Varieties of Religious Experience.* London: Longmans, Green.

Mayer-Gross, W. 1935. On Depersonalization. *Brit. J. Med. Psych.* 15:103-26.

Noyes, R., Jr. 1972. "The Experience of Dying." *Psychiatry* 35:174-84.

Noyes, R., and R. Kletii. In press. Depersonalization in the Face of Life-Threatening Danger: An Interpretation. *Omega.*

Schilder, P. 1928. *Introduction to a Psychoanalytic Psychiatry.* Nervous and Mental Disease Publ.

Slater, E., and M. Roth. 1969. *Clinical Psychiatry.* 3rd ed. London: Williams and Wilkins.

Stace, W.T. 1960. *Mysticism and Philosophy.* New York: Lippincott.

5

Deathbed Observations by Physicians and Nurses: A Cross-Cultural Survey

Karlis Osis and Erlendur Haraldsson

INTRODUCTION

AT TIMES DYING PATIENTS "SEE" PERSONS AND visionary landscapes which others present do not see. Usually such deathbed visions are interpreted as mere hallucinations which have no basis in external reality. In the early years of psychical research, Myers (1903) and Hyslop (1908) recognized some possibly paranormal elements in a few selected cases of visions of dying patients. Sir William Barrett, a physicist of the Royal College of Science, Dublin, was interested in such cases and presented a number of them in a small book entitled *Death-Bed Visions* (1926). While some of his cases were carefully observed by physicians and nurses, others are of lesser evidential quality. Barrett was particularly impressed by visions that seemed to mirror some form of contact between patients who were fully rational and cognizant of their physical surroundings and their deceased relatives who, presumably, had passed on to the "other world." Often in these cases the ostensible purpose of the deceased was to take the patient away to a post-mortem plane of existence. Barrett emphasized cases in which apparitions ran contrary to the patient's expectations, for example, apparitions of persons the patient thought were still living, but who in fact were dead. In several of Barrett's cases the apparitions were experienced either with exalted feelings or with emotions of serenity and peace. Deathbed visions, Barrett pointed out, often did not conform to cultural stereotypes, e.g., dying children were surprised to see "angels" without wings.

Some 30 years later, Barrett's work inspired one of us (K.O.) to systematically study deathbed experiences using modern survey methods and statistical evaluations. In 1959-60, under the auspices of the Parapsychology Foundation, K.O. conducted such a survey. It was the first of its kind and will be referred to in this paper as the "pilot survey." The report on the pilot survey was published by the Parapsychology Foundation as a monograph, *Deathbed Observations by Physicians and Nurses* (Osis 1961).

K.O. found that deathbed visions which appear to be suggestive of post-mortem survival tended to be independent of factors known to cause hallucinations, enhance their occurrence, or influence their content. Medical factors—such as illness predisposing to hallucinatory experiences, high fevers, medication with morphine, etc.—did not seem to generate an increase in the frequency of after-life related experiences. In some instances, such medical factors even appeared to suppress survival-related phenomena. Moreover, personal variables such as the patient's sex, age, education, socio-economic status, and religious affiliation also appeared to be of little importance.

The contents of the dying patients' hallucinations were analyzed and found to be different from those of hallucinations in the general population and the mentally ill. For example, hallucinations of the dying are usually visual, as is the case in most ESP experiences, and rarely auditory, the predominant mode in mentally disturbed persons. Terminal patients were reported to have seen apparitions of the deceased, rather than of the living, two or three times more often than do people in the general population. Of all the apparitions of identified persons, 90% were of relatives of the patient; of these, 90% were close relatives: mother, father, spouse, sibling, and offspring. This occurs infrequently in the hallucinations of the general population.

K.O. also performed extensive interaction analyses on the data of the pilot study. This led to the discovery of many patterns which supported the post-mortem survival hypothesis. He believed, however, since most of the findings were post hoc, that without verification in later surveys the weight of the findings would be rather limited.

The two new cross-cultural surveys described in this paper were carried out to replicate the pilot study. The range of questions was greatly expanded in order to obtain more information which might either support the evidence for post-mortem survival, or provide facts contradicting it and thus lend weight to what we have termed the "destruction hypothesis." Information from the pilot survey and other sources was used to formulate a model, or series of hypotheses concerning deathbed visions. The model is a bi-polar one which sharply contrasts two mutually exclusive concepts: the survival hypothesis and the destruction hypothesis.

A Model of the Two Basic Hypotheses of Deathbed Visions

Survival	*Destruction*
Death is the transition to another mode of existence.	Death is the ultimate destruction of the personality.

A. Sources of Deathbed Visions

Extrasensory Perception	*Sick Brain or Delusions*
1. Extrasensory awareness of discarnate entities, e.g., deceased relatives and religious figures.	1. Malfunction of the nervous system and the dying brain.
2. Clairvoyant or precognitive glimpses of post-mortem existence.	2. Schizoid reactions to severe stress.

B. Influence of Hallucinogenic Factors on Deathbed Visions

Independent of Medical Factors	*Dependent on Medical Factors*
1. The presence of hallucinogenic medical factors will not increase the frequency of visions related to post-mortem existence.	1. The presence of hallucinogenic medical factors will increase the frequency of hallucinations related to post-mortem existence—i.e.,

the more disturbed the brain processes, the more numerous the "otherworld" fantasies.

2. Conditions detrimental to ESP will decrease the frequency of after-life related phenomena.

2. ESP not involved.

C. Content of Deathbed Visions

Perceptions	Hallucinations
1. After-life related visions will be relatively coherent, and oriented to the situation of dying and the transition to another mode of existence, including "otherworldly" messengers and environments.	1. Hallucinations will portray only memories already stored in the brain and express desires, expectations, and fears of the individual, as well as beliefs characteristic of his culture.

D. Influence of Psychological Factors on Deathbed Visions

Conditions Related to Awareness of an "Other World"	Conditions Related to Hallucinations of This World or "Other-World" Fantasies
1. Clarity of consciousness and an intact sense of reality will facilitate awareness of an "other world" and its messengers, while states in which contact with external reality is absent will impair such awareness.	1. Clarity of consciousness and an intact sense of reality will be less conducive to all kinds of hallucinations than states in which contact with reality is absent.
2. Patients' expectation of recovery or dying will not influence the occurrence of after-life related visions.	2. Patients' expectation of recovery will facilitate this-life hallucinations, while expectation of dying will facilitate hallucinations of an after-life.
3. Presence of stress will not increase the frequency of visions related to an after-life.	3. Presence of stress will increase the frequency of hallucinations related to an after-life.

E. Variability of Content Across Individuals and Cultures

Perceptions	Hallucinations
1. Little variability.	1. Much variability.
2. Visions involving basic characteristics of the "other world" will be essentially similar for men and women, young and old, educated and illiterate, religious and nonreligious, Christian and Hindu, American and Indian. Only minor differences among them will be expected.	2. Hallucinations are purely subjective. They will vary widely with the dispositions, psychological dynamics, and cultural background of the individual.

METHOD

We approached physicians and nurses in both the United States and India in two steps: (a) a two-page initial questionnaire was distributed concerning the extent and kinds of observations they had made of dying patients, and of those who were close to death but recovered; (b) individual interviews were held with respondents on the details of cases reported in the questionnaires and which fell within the scope of the survey.

Questionnaires and Procedure

The survey in the U.S. was conducted between 1961 and 1964 in New York, New Jersey, Connecticut, Rhode Island, and Pennsylvania. The second survey was carried out in Northern India during 1972-73.

Although the same basic questionnaire was used in both surveys, slight adjustments were made in the questions asked of the Indian respondents—e.g., tropical diseases and the Hindu and Moslem religions were covered—in order to accommodate them to the cultural differences.

In the initial questionnaire we asked the medical personnel about their observations of the following:

1. Hallucinations of *human figures* experienced by (a) *terminal* patients (those not recovering), and (b) by *non-terminal* patients (those who were close to death but recovered).

2. Hallucinations of *surroundings* (landscapes, etc.) experienced by (a) *terminal* patients, and (b) by *non-terminal* patients.

3. Mood elevation (sudden rise of mood to elation or serenity) in *terminal* patients.

In the U.S. the questionnaire, with a covering letter, was mailed to a stratified random sample of 2500 physicians and 2500 nurses. Those not responding received another letter asking for a reply. A total of 1004 responses was received.

Our Indian consultants advised us not to use the mails to distribute the questionnaire. We therefore worked mainly in large university hospitals. Usually the professor of medicine or professor of surgery arranged meetings with the hospital staff during which we gave a short talk and distributed the questionnaires to be filled out. Practically all the physicians and nurses we approached returned the completed questionnaires (a total of 704).

Interviews

American respondents who reported pertinent cases were interviewed by telephone. In India, telephone contacts had to be replaced by personal interviews, mainly in hospitals but sometimes in the homes of the respondents.

We developed three separate follow-up questionnaires for the following types of experience: (a) hallucinations of human figures, (b) hallucinations of surroundings, and (c) mood elevation. Each of these questionnaires consisted of 69 questions used to guide the interview.

Open-ended questions were used, e.g., "What was the patient's behavior indicating that he/she was experiencing hallucinations?" Questions proposing a set of alternative answers were also used, e.g., "Was the patient calmed by the hallucination, did he/she become excited, or was there no apparent effect?"

Questions covered (a) characteristics of the patient such as sex, age, education, religious belief and degree of involvement in it, and belief in an after-life; and (b) medical factors such as diagnosis, medical history, medication, temperature, and clarity of consciousness. Additional questions elicited information from the respondents concerning their date of graduation from professional school, degree received, religious beliefs, belief in life after death, and attitudes toward hallucinations. The main part of the questionnaire was devoted to obtaining as many details as possible about the experience reported, e.g., how the patient described the hallucination. A total of 877 cases, about evenly divided between the U.S. and India, comprise the main part of the data.

Evaluation of the Data

The interview data were coded and recorded on computer cards. Each item in the various categories was analyzed for frequency of occurrence. For example, responses to the question, "What was the primary diagnosis of the illness?" were grouped into basic categories such as malignancies, cardiovascular disease, respiratory disease, kidney disease, brain disease or injury, etc. Then the data were submitted to cross-tabulations. Items describing factors that might influence each other were considered jointly: for example, comparisons between the number of patients suffering from diseases known to cause hallucinations (brain diseases, uremia) and the number of patients suffering from other kinds of diseases were made in terms of the frequency with which the patients hallucinated living persons, dead persons, etc. Differences were assessed by chi-square statistics. We report below only probabilities associated with the chi-square analyses. We used the significance level of $P = .05$ (two-tailed).

RESULTS

We completed a similar number of interviews in the U.S. (442) and in India (435). The vast majority of patients involved were terminally ill (714). We also had 163 cases of patients who recovered from near-death conditions. Hallucinations of human figures, or seeing apparitions, was the type of phenomenon most frequently reported (by 591 patients). A total of 112 vision cases were primarily of heavenly abodes, landscapes, gardens, buildings. In 174 cases, patients did not report seeing anything unusual, but their moods became elevated to serenity, peace, elation, or religious emotions. This report covers only cases of apparitions of human figures seen by terminal patients (471 cases).

Characteristics of Apparitions Seen
by Terminal Patients

As noted above, reports of terminal patients "seeing" persons not observed by others present comprise by far the largest and most interesting part of our data. The sample derives from 216 interviews with American respondents and 255 from Indian respondents.

Duration of Apparition. As in most instances of spontaneous ESP, the apparitional experiences were usually of quite brief duration: 48% lasted for five minutes or less, 17% from six to 15 minutes, and only 17% for more than an hour (Table 1, Row a).

Timing of Apparition. The closer in time the apparition was to the patient's death (Table 1, Row b), the more frequently it had characteristics suggestive of an after-life. The time between seeing an apparition and losing consciousness was generally shorter than the time between losing consciousness and clinical death.

Identity of Apparition. The apparitions in our sample portrayed living persons, dead persons, and mythological or historical religious figures. According to the findings of the pilot study, apparitions of the living have nothing to do with post-mortem survival. On the other hand, apparitions of the dead and of religious figures may have characteristics suggestive of life after death. We termed apparitions in this category "survival-related apparitions," and they comprised 80% of the cases in the pilot survey. The proportion of survival-related apparitions in the present survey was remarkably similar to that of the pilot survey: 83% in the U.S. and 79% in India (Table 1, Row c).

Could these proportions be characteristic of hallucinations in general among persons who are not near death? Fortunately, two British surveys of hallucinations experienced by the general population provided data for comparison. In the "Census of Hallucinations" (H. Sidgwick and Committee 1894) it was reported that only 33% of the sample had hallucinations similar to those in our survival-related group; D.J. West (1948, p. 190) reported 22% in a "mass observation" survey. (Categories that do not fit our classification scheme are excluded in the calculation of these percentages.) Thus we conclude that terminal patients in both the pilot and in the present survey saw apparitions of the dead and of religious figures about three times more frequently than the general population sampled in these two British studies.

While the proportion of survival-related apparitions in the U.S. and India is remarkably stable, the identity of the apparitions experienced within this group varied greatly. American patients for the most part saw deceased persons while Indian patients predominantly saw religious figures (Table 1, Row c; Table 2, Rows a and b). In a detailed analysis to be reported elsewhere we were able to trace

TABLE 1

Characteristics of the Apparitional Experience in Terminal Patients

Variables	Characteristics	Number of Cases			Percentage*		
		U.S.	India	Total	U.S.	India	Total
a. Duration of	1 sec.-5 min.	85	83	168	65	38	48
apparition	6-15 min.	17	43	60	13	20	17
	16-59 min.	11	50	61	9	23	18
	1 hr.-1 day	13	31	44	10	14	13
	Longer	4	10	14	3	5	4
	No information	86	38	124	—	—	—
b. Interval between	0-10 min.	17	36	53	9	14	12
apparition and	11-59 min.	7	59	66	4	23	15
death	1-6 hrs.	26	64	90	13	25	20
	7-24 hrs.	28	41	69	14	17	15
	Longer	117	52	169	60	21	38
	No information	21	3	24	—	—	—
c. Identity of	Living	30	38	68	16	20	18
apparition	Dead	124	54	178	66	28	47
	Religious figure	22	93	115	12	48	30
	Combination of above	11	7	18	6	4	5
	No information	29	63	92	—	—	—
d. Sex of apparition	Male	59	103	162	39	77	57
	Female	91	30	121	61	23	43
	No information	66	122	188	—	—	—
e. Purpose of	Taken for visitor	14	28	42	14	14	14
apparition	To comfort patient	13	4	17	13	2	6
	To take patient away, with consent	40	102	142	41	50	47
	To take patient away, without consent	1	53	54	1	26	18
	To send patient back	0	2	2	0	1	1
	Threatening	4	13	17	4	6	6
	Reliving memories	26	1	27	27	1	9
	No information	118	52	170	—	—	—
f. Emotional reactions,	No effect or relaxation	60	65	125	31	28	30
1st group	Serenity	46	40	86	23	18	20
	Elation	56	32	88	29	14	21
	Negative	33	91	124	17	40	29
	No information	21	27	48	—	—	—
g. Emotional reactions	No effect or relaxation	60	65	125	31	28	30
2nd group	Negative	33	91	124	17	40	29
	Positive, nonreligious	77	36	113	39	16	27
	Positive, religious	25	36	61	13	16	14
	No information	21	27	48	—	—	—

*Percentages do not include cases about which no information was available. Figures in some percentage columns do not add up to 100 due to rounding off.

some, but not all, of the reasons which might account for these differences. In the visions of the Indian patients (especially the males), female figures were extremely rare (Table 1, Row d). This fact alone could have reduced the total number of apparitions of the dead, thereby increasing the proportion of religious figures in the Indian sample (Table 2, Row b). Thus, while the frequency of survival-related apparitions is the same in both samples, the characteristics of these apparitions are strongly molded by cultural forces.

Ninety-one percent of all identified apparitions of persons were relatives of the patient. (In 20%, the identity of the apparition was not ascertained.) Of these, 90% were close relatives, i.e., mother, spouse, offspring, sibling, and father—in that order of frequency (Table 2, Row a). The religious figures were usually described merely as an angel or god, or were unidentified. When identified they were named according to the patient's religion, e.g., no Hindu reported seeing Jesus; no Christian a Hindu deity.

Purpose of Apparition. Quite often patients told respondents why the apparition had visited them. In 50% of the cases in the pilot survey, the stated purpose of the apparition was to aid patients in their transition to another world: "to take them away." In the present study this purpose was reported in 65% of the cases (Table 1, Row e). For further analyses we excluded two somewhat ambiguous categories: that the figure came "to comfort" the patient, which could imply either a "this-life" purpose or a "take-away" purpose, and cases where patients were said to be "reliving memories" which, of course, indicates no contemporary purposes. Thus, after adjusting the data in this way, the take-away purpose is clearly dominant in all three surveys: pilot, 76%; U.S., 69%; India, 79%.

Patients' Response to Apparition. In the pilot survey it was found that a large majority (89%) of the patients who saw apparitions with a take-away purpose eagerly consented "to go" with them. Although consent was expressed in 72% of the present survey's take-away cases, 28% did not consent, and some patients reacted with fright and screams for help. Practically all these negative responses came from Indian patients who refused to consent (Table 1, Row e). In our unpublished interaction analyses we found that this difference in consent between the U.S. and Indian samples may be partly due to the patients' religion and partly to their nationality.

TABLE 2

Identity of Apparitional Figures*

Variables	Identity	U.S.	India	Total	U.S.	India	Total
			Number of Figures			Percentage**	
	Mother	60	16	76	28	14	23
	Father	15	16	31	7	14	9
	Spouse	49	10	59	23	8	18
	Sibling	27	15	42	12	13	13
	Offspring	27	17	44	12	14	13
	Other relatives, previous generation	5	7	12	2	6	4
a. Secular	Other relatives, same generation	2	10	12	1	8	4
	Other relatives, next generation	0	4	4	0	3	1
	Unidentified relatives	9	14	23	4	12	7
	Friends, acquaintances	21	8	29	10	7	9
	Unidentified persons	25	61	86	—	—	—
	Totals:	240	178	418	—	—	—
	God or Jesus	13	17	30	42	22	28
	Shiva, Rama, Krishna	0	13	13	0	17	12
	Mary, Kali, Durga	5	4	9	16	5	8
	God of death & messengers	0	18	18	0	24	17
b. Religious	Saints & gurus	3	5	8	10	7	8
	Angels, Devi, etc.	9	17	26	29	22	24
	Demons & devils	1	2	3	3	3	3
	Other religious figures, unidentified	2	31	33	—	—	—
	Totals:	33	107	140	—	—	—

*Totals include cases in which several figures were seen by the same patient.
**Percentages do not include cases about which no information was available. Figures in some percentage columns do not add up to 100 due to rounding off.

Patients were said to have reacted to the apparition with noticeable emotions in 70% of the cases.[2] Many of them reacted with positive emotions (41%), while a considerable number (29%) had negative emotions—particularly in cases where the patient did not consent "to go" with the apparition. Of those with positive emotional reactions, half were serene and peaceful and half were elated (Table 1, Row f). We also asked our respondents to evaluate patients' positive emotions as religious or nonreligious feelings (Table 1, Row g). They reported that 35% of those positive emotions were of religious nature. Terminal patients usually suffer from pain and other kinds of discomfort; consequently their moods are rather depressed. The elation and serenity that the survival-related apparitions aroused in most of the patients contrasted sharply against the gloom of dying.

Medical Factors

Drugs. Various medical factors are known to increase the likeliood of hallucinatory behavior. Medication consisting of certain analgesics and sedatives, such as morphine and Demerol, might have caused hallucinations in some of our cases. However, the majority (61%) of the 425 patients about whom we have such information had not received drugs which could cause hallucinations. Half of those who were under sedation had received such small doses or such weak drugs that the respondents did not consider them to have been psychologically affected. Of the 20% who were influenced, more than half (11%) were said to be only mildly affected. Eight percent were moderately affected and only 1% strongly affected (Table 3, Row d). Thus the evidence indicates that in most cases the apparitional experiences were not drug-induced.

Temperature. High body temperature sometimes leads to hallucinations. Only 8% of the patients ran fevers of over 103 degrees (measured orally) which might have facilitated hallucinatory behavior (Table 3, Row c).

Diagnoses. Hallucinations may be associated with injury and diseases of the brain, and with uremic poisoning caused by kidney malfunction, although many brain-injured patients, especially those with strokes, do not hallucinate. Only 12% of the patients in our sample, including stroke cases, had such diagnoses (Table 3, Row a).

In addition to primary diagnoses, we also considered secondary illnesses, previous illnesses, and any other factors in the patient's history which might have been hallucinogenic, e.g., alcoholism or mental illness. This measure is rather inflated since we included in it diagnoses only suspected by the physician and diseases which were not active at the time of the terminal illness. We also included the primary diagnoses involving the three hallucinogenic categories discussed above. Only 25% of the patients had secondary diagnoses which could have been hallucinogenic (Table 3, Row b).

"Hallucinogenic Index." It was also important to know how many patients might have had at least one of the following possible hallucinogenic factors: drugs, high fever, and primary and/or secondary diagnoses of a hallucinogenic nature. We therefore established a "hallucinogenic index" which includes every patient who had one or more of the above-mentioned indices. It should be noted that we included in this index cases which do not strongly suggest that the patients' hallucinations were of an abnormal origin, e.g., stroke cases, cases in which medication only slightly affected clarity of consciousness, etc. Nevertheless, such indices are present in only 38% of the cases; the majority (62%) are free of them. In the pilot survey, it was found that deathbed visions are relatively unaffected by medical factors. The data from the present survey give the same impression.

Clarity of Consciousness. We inquired into the clarity of consciousness of the patient at the time of the apparitional experience, a condition which is closely related to medical factors. We had this information for 457 cases. Almost half (43%) the patients were in a normal state of consciousness; they were fully aware of and responsive to their environment. In 29% awareness was mildly impaired, but the respondents could still communicate with their patients. Only 17% were in such a severely impaired state of consciousness that little or no communication was possible. In 11% clarity fluctuated and could not be accurately determined for the times the hallucinations were experienced (Table 3, Row e).

Hallucinogenic medical factors are clearly absent in two-thirds of our data. Could these factors nevertheless have affected the remaining third of the patients who were included in the "hallucinogenic index"? Could they have spuriously enhanced the frequency of those characteristics which were found in the pilot study to support the post-mortem survival hypothesis? These characteristics are (a) predominance of survival-related apparitions of dead persons and religious figures, (b) their "take-away" purpose, and (c) the patients' appropriate emotional reactions. Cross-tabulations between the "hallucinogenic index" and the nature of the apparition (living, dead, or religious figure) show that there was no significant interaction. The presence of hallucinogenic factors did not increase the frequency of survival-related trends such as apparitions of the deceased, religious figures, or expression of the "take-away" purpose. Hallucinogenic factors did, however, significantly affect

TABLE 3

Medical Status of Terminal Patients Seeing Apparitions

Variables	Medical Status	Number of Patients U.S.	India	Total	Percentage* U.S.	India	Total
a. Primary diagnosis	Cancer	79	28	107	37	11	23
	Heart & circulatory disease	61	39	100	29	16	22
	Injury & post-operative	10	62	72	5	25	16
	Respiratory disease	9	26	35	4	11	8
	Brain injury/disease, uremia	28	26	54	13	11	12
	Miscellaneous	25	64	89	12	26	19
	No information	4	10	14	—	—	—
b. Secondary diagnosis, possibly hallucinogenic	Present	68	40	108	33	18	25
	Absent	137	187	324	67	82	75
	No information	11	28	39	—	—	—
c. Body temperature (oral)	Less than 100°	128	129	257	64	53	58
	100°-103°	55	94	149	28	39	34
	Above 103°	16	20	36	8	8	8
	No information	17	12	29	—	—	—
d. Medication affecting consciousness	None	94	165	259	49	71	61
	Medication, no effect	39	40	79	20	17	19
	Mildly affected	31	18	49	16	8	11
	Moderately affected	22	10	32	12	4	8
	Strongly affected	5	1	6	3	0	1
	No information	25	21	46	—	—	—
e. Clarity of consciousness	Clear	98	100	198	48	39	43
	Mildly impaired	31	103	134	15	41	29
	Severely impaired	36	39	75	18	15	17
	Fluctuating	38	12	50	19	5	11
	No information	13	1	14	—	—	—

*Percentages do not include cases about which no information was available.

the expected emotional reactions of the patients in the American sample ($P = .03$). They seemed to suppress serenity, peace, and religious emotions, and to increase the incidence of negative reactions. This trend is not significant in the Indian sample. We conclude that the medical variables ascertained in the survey seem to be relatively unrelated to the apparitional experiences in terminal patients.

Demographic Factors

Demographic factors such as age, sex, educational and occupation (Table 4, Rows a-d) did not interact significantly with any aspects of the patients' apparitional experiences.

Psychological Factors

We analyzed several psychological factors to determine whether they tended to shape the phenomenological aspects of the main phenomena: apparitions of the living, the dead, and religious figures; purpose of the apparitions; and the patients' emotional reactions to them.

Stress. Hallucinations tend to occur in situations of severe stress and social deprivation (Siegel and L.J. West 1976; L.J. West 1962). Not only are visits to terminal patients by relatives and friends often restricted, but most such patients are going through very stressful situations, compounded by having to cope with severe pain. Therefore, could their hallucinatory experiences be due to stress rather than to extrasensory awareness of "visitors" from another mode of existence? We attempted to answer this question by evaluating an indirect indication of stress found in the data of the patients in our sample—their mood on the day before the hallucination occurred. We assumed that negative moods such as anxiety, anger, or depression would indicate more stress than would positive moods. The least stress, we believed, would be indicated by moods designated by our respondents as "normal" or "average."

There were no significant interactions between the patients' moods on the day prior to the apparitional experiences and what the apparition represented. We also failed to find any appreciable interaction between the mood and patients' emotional reactions to the apparitional experience. The purpose of the apparition was not significantly related to mood in either the American or the Indian sample taken separately. However, this relationship is significant in the pooled data from both populations ($P = .001$), and it is in the direction opposite to what would be expected on the hypothesis that stress is a causative factor in apparitional experiences. Patients with normal moods experienced apparitions with a peaceful "take-away" purpose more frequently (54%) than did those who had positive (31%) or negative (27%) moods. From these data we may infer that while the stress experienced by the terminal patients might have caused other kinds of hallucinations, it is unlikely that it affected the incidence of apparitions which expressed purposes related to post-mortem survival.

Desires and Expectations. A patient's desires, expectations, or "wishful thinking" might be possible causes of hallucinations. For example, a thirsty traveler in the desert might have the illusion of seeing water when none was there. We ascertained from our respondents the number of patients who had expressed a desire to have a visit from a living person, such as a spouse or a child, and then checked on how many of these persons were later hallucinated. We found only 13 such cases, an insignificant fraction of the total sample. Furthermore, there were no indications in the data to suggest that persons who had recently visited the patient appeared frequently in his hallucinations. Of those visitors, only nine were hallucinated.

Fear of Dying. In order to cope with their fear of dying, patients who expect to die might be motivated to hallucinate "messengers" from the after-life. (This would not be the case for patients who expect to recover.) In neither the American nor the Indian sample, however, were the intentions or identity of the survival-related apparitions significantly correlated with the patients' expectations of living or dying. This is particularly apparent in cases where the patient did not consent to the "take-away" purpose of the apparition and screamed for help. Patients' emotional reactions to the apparitional experiences also failed to relate significantly to the motivational variables ascertained in the surveys.

Cultural Factors

We hoped that cross-cultural comparisons would throw light on the hypothesis that some deathbed visions may portray certain aspects of a reality external to the patient.

According to our model we assume that some apparitions may in some way exist independent of the observer. As cultural factors have a more powerful effect on subjective hallucinatory experiences than on observations of external reality, the degree of influence of such factors as religion and belief in post-mortem survival might give a clue as to the true nature of deathbed visions.

TABLE 4

Characteristics of Terminal Patients Seeing Apparitions

Variables	Characteristics	Number of Patients			Percentage*		
		U.S.	India	Total	U.S.	India	Total
a. Age	1-30	19	68	87	9	27	19
	31-50	22	97	119	10	38	25
	Over 50	174	90	264	81	35	56
	No information	1	0	1	—	—	—
b. Sex	Male	99	175	274	46	69	58
	Female	117	80	197	54	31	42
c. Education	None, pre-school	13	77	90	7	32	21
	Primary	57	59	116	30	25	27
	High school	73	65	138	39	27	32
	College	45	38	83	24	16	20
	No information	28	16	44	—	—	—
d. Occupation	Professional, manager, clergy	56	29	85	41	19	30
	Clerical, sales, crafts	9	40	49	7	26	17
	Farmer, laborer, services, housewife	70	83	153	52	55	53
	No information	81	103	184	—	—	—
e. Religion	Hindu	—	214	214	—	85	48
	Christian	—	26	26	—	10	6
	Moslem	—	12	12	—	5	3
	Protestant	97	—	97	51	—	22
	Catholic	68	—	68	36	—	15
	Jewish	12	—	12	6	—	3
	Other or none	14	—	14	7	—	3
	No information	25	3	28	—	—	—
f. Degree of involvement in religion	No involvement	12	3	15	8	2	5
	Slight	27	12	39	18	9	14
	Moderate	44	48	92	30	38	33
	Deep	64	65	129	44	51	47
	No information	69	127	196	—	—	—
g. Belief in an after-life	Belief	69	70	139	92	92	92
	No belief	6	6	12	8	8	8
	No information	141	179	320	—	—	—

*Percentages do not include cases about which no information was available. Figures in some percentage columns do not add up to 100 due to rounding off.

Religion. Our sample population consisted mainly of Christians (43%) and Hindus (48%). In the U.S. the stratifications were 51% Protestant, 36% Catholic, 6% Jewish, and 7% unaffiliated or belonging to other religions. Eighty-five percent of the Indian patients were Hindu, 10% were Christian, and 5% were Moslem (Table 4, Row e). This distribution roughly equals the affiliation proportions among the general population in the areas surveyed, except for the small unaffiliated group in the U.S. This discrepancy disappears if we assume that most of the patients whose affiliations were not reported actually were not affiliated with any religious denomination. Apparently religious affiliation was not a factor in determining the phenomena. The question remains, however, whether the patients' religion could have determined the important core characteristics of the apparitions. Religion did not significantly influence the purpose or the kind of apparition seen (living, dead, or religious figures). And both the occurrences of survival-related apparitions (of the dead and/or religious figures) and their after-life purposes appear to have transcended the widely divergent religious ideologies of Hindus, Catholics, Protestants, Jews, and Moslems.

The patients' emotional reactions of serenity, elation, and religious feelings engendered by apparitional experiences were similar among Catholics and Protestants in the U.S. Unfortunately, we had too few patients of other religions for effective comparison in the American sample. Therefore Catholics and Protestants were compared only with the rest of the patients as a whole—including those who were unaffiliated, those of other religions, and those whose affiliations were not reported. This mixed group showed different emotional reactions such as less serenity ($P = .02$) and less religions feelings. ($P = .06$).

In India the small minority of Christian patients was reported to have reacted more with serenity and religious emotion than the Hindus did. Part of this difference was traced to the respondent bias of Christian nurses and therefore it cannot be interpreted with reasonable certainty. However, there were more similarities than differences: like Americans, many Hindu patients responded with serenity, peace, and religious emotions.

The real difference between the American and Indian reactions to the apparitional experience lies in the patients' readiness to consent to the "take-away" purpose of the apparition: with only one exception, all the American patients were ready "to go," while 34%

of the Indian patients were not. Can this be explained in terms of their differences in religion? There was indeed a difference, though not a significant one: only 16% of the Indian Christians did not consent "to go," as compared to 37% of the Hindu patients. It seems probable that this no-consent attitude is due to both national and religious factors. Patients' involvement in religion did not significantly affect the nature of the apparition experienced, its purpose, or their emotional reactions to it.

Belief in Life after Death. A patient's belief in life after death is important for understanding his ways of coping with approaching death. Yet surprisingly few (one third) of our respondents were aware of their patients' beliefs, or lack thereof, in an after-life. The majority of them reported that they either did not discuss the matter with the patients, or did not pay enough attention to remember it (68% of the cases). It is remarkable that 12 patients who *did not* believe in life after death saw apparitions (Table 4, Row g). This, of course, is too small a sample for detailed interaction analysis. We assumed that patients whose beliefs were weak or non-existent might have been more likely to neglect mentioning the matter to their physicians or nurses than would those who had strong convictions. We therefore contrasted this "no information" group with the believers.

Our analysis revealed that belief in an after-life has no significant influence on the frequency of the kind of apparition seen, though it did seem to influence the patient's ostensible communication with it. More patients in the "believers" group than those in the "no information" group experienced apparitions with a "take away" purpose and consented "to go" with them. This difference is significant in both the U.S. ($P = .05$) and the Indian ($P = .004$) sample. There was no such difference in Indian patients who did not consent "to go." (Since there was only one "non-consenter" in the American sample, this comparison could not be made.)

Belief in life after death did not significantly affect serenity and elation in the American patients, but it did increase such feelings at the expense of negative reactions in the Indian sample ($P = .005$). In both countries, belief strongly increased positive religious responses (U.S., $P = .004$; India, $P = .002$).

A number of other variables were ascertained and analyzed— among them the possibility of respondent bias, as mentioned above—but they are not discussed here due to lack of space. Reports of phenomena other than hallucinations of human figures were also collected and evaluated: visions of scenery, etc., mood elevation shortly before death, and experiences of patients who were near death but recovered. We hope to report on these elsewhere.

DISCUSSION

The American and Indian surveys were designed to replicate the findings of the pilot survey and to provide more detailed data bearing on the hypothesis of post-mortem survival. While the pilot survey unearthed many findings which were interpreted as being consistent with the after-life hypothesis, it had severe limitations concerning the statistical certainty of these findings. Because the pilot survey was the first of its kind, previous information was inadequate in helping to predict many of the trends which emerged in that study. Therefore the possibility that such unexpected trends were due to chance variations could not be ruled out. However, most trends in the present survey are reasonably consistent among themselves and with those of the pilot survey. This diminishes the probability of chance as an acceptable explanation.

Our model of deathbed experiences related to post-mortem survival assumes (a) that survival-oriented apparitions may to some extent be due to ESP of or from "another world" (e.g., deceased relatives or religious figures) or (b), if this is not the case, are entirely subjective. Therefore we hypothesized that medical factors which often cause hallucinations but which are not known to affect ESP will not increase the frequency of seeing after-life related apparitions. In all three surveys, the data conformed to this hypothesis. Furthermore, we postulated that medical conditions which impede sensory (and, we presume, extrasensory) contact with the external world also reduce the incidence of seeing after-life oriented hallucinations. This was confirmed.

We carefully considered psychological factors which might have caused hallucinations. Severe stress, especially in situations of drastically reduced social contact, can find release in hallucinations. Psychiatrists suggest that deathbed visions actually are schizoid episodes through which patients cope with very stressful situations by hallucinating pleasing fantasies of another world. A careful analysis of the data revealed no support for this counterhypothesis. Stress was not significantly related to the core phenomena of deathbed visions. In both the American and Indian samples, the trend went in the opposite direction: stress tended to reduce the survival-related aspects of these experiences. Patients' desires, wishes, and expectations also had no significant influence. In a large number of cases, patients experienced apparitions which appeared to be in opposition to their own motivations, though consistent with our hypothesis of post-mortem survival. Some psychiatrists have developed the concept of "latent motivation"—motivation which is not expressed verbally or exhibited in behavior. However, this concept has been severely criticized and generally rejected in scientific research. We did not find any definite indices in our data of "latent motivation" with regard to the main phenomena of deathbed visions.

The most viable counterhypothesis is cultural conditioning. In childhood and youth, cultural beliefs are transmitted to us in various ways. Could they re-emerge in the visions of the dying—a kind of playing back of old records? The cross-cultural survey in India was primarily done with this question in view. Our model assumes that individual and cultural factors will completely shape deathbed visions, provided they are *caused* by these factors. However, if they are based on perception of some form of external reality, or ESP glimpses of "another world," we hypothesized that only modest differences between cultures would emerge, with the main features remaining the same. An analogy could be found by contrasting a typically American and a typically Indian painting of a mountain: the details would be quite different while the basic characteristics of a mountain would be clearly recognizable.

We found a very close agreement in all three surveys with regard to the frequencies of survival-related apparitions: dead and religious figures versus those of the living. The ostensible "take-away" purpose of the apparition was also equally present. Absence of influences by medical and psychological variables was indicated in all three samples. The core phenomena are the same.

Cultural coloring, however, was present. The sex of the hallucinatory figure was largely determined by culturally conditioned preferences which, in turn, seem to influence the proportion of hallucinations of dead and religious figures. Religion had a comparably slight influence on the main phenomena, though it did, of course, determine the naming of the religious figures. We interpret these modest cultural differences according to our model:

they seem to support the hypothesis that deathbed visions are, in part, based on extrasensory perception of some form of external reality rather than having entirely subjective origins.

Each culture develops dominant attitudes or values concerning what is desirable and meritorious to say or do, and what is undesirable and degrading. In Western culture, talking about personal contact with the dead is often felt to be undesirable. In spite of the fact that 27% of an American sample studied by Greeley (1975) answered "yes" to the question "Have you ever felt that you were really in touch with someone who had died?" only rarely were such experiences told to professional people. In a British survey, Rees (1971) contacted 277 widows and 66 widowers in selected localities. Of this number, 94% were suitable for interview. Forty-seven percent of that sample reported hallucinations of the presence of a dead spouse. None of them discussed their experiences with their doctors, and only one out of 137 did so with a clergyman. The main reason for not discussing the experience was fear of ridicule. It is likely that patients in our survey also had a negative response bias; that is, they avoided telling medical personnel about "seeing" apparitions of the dead. If this is so, our sample represents fewer survival-related apparitions than the number actually experienced.

Another possible way in which cultural conditioning could shape the data is through respondent bias. The medical observers might have reported what they believed they were supposed to, according to cultural norms, and left out what went against the grain of their particular culture. We found no serious distortion in favor of the after-life hypothesis. On the contrary, we detected some under-reporting of those phenomena which we hypothesize as being related to post-mortem survival.

Our data came from interviews with physicians and nurses rather than with the patients themselves. This could introduce a source of bias in reporting and sampling. However, some studies by Moody and Kübler-Ross are based upon interviews with patients. In Moody's (1975) account of the experiences of resuscitated patients, he states that quite a few of these patients, while in a near-death state, became aware of the presence of deceased relatives as well as what we have called religious figures "who apparently were there to ease them through their transition to death" (p. 43). In a personal communication Kübler-Ross (1976) has on the basis of her experience with terminal patients confirmed the main characteristics of our own findings: a predominance of survival-related apparitions, their "take-away" purpose, and patients' reactions of serenity, peace, and religious emotion.

The issue of survival after death obviously cannot be assessed solely on the basis of experiences of dying patients. The entire range of other phenomena suggestive of an after-life—such as out-of-body experiences, reincarnation memories, apparitions collectively perceived, and certain kinds of mediumistic communications—have to be considered together with the various explanatory hypotheses (other than survival) that have been advanced (see, e.g., Hart, 1956, 1959; Murphy, 1961; Roll, 1974; E.M. Sidgwick, 1923; Stevenson, 1974a, 1974b, 1975; Tyrrell, 1953). Noyes (1972), Noyes and Kletti (1972, 1976), and Garfield (1975) have published surveys of cases which involve deathbed experiences characterized by altered states, panoramic memories, and also some phenomena similar to those covered in the present report, but without having ascribed to them an after-life interpretation. Discussion of the full range of data and theories related to the survival question does not fall into the scope of this paper.

We conclude our report on the cross-cultural survey of the experiences of dying patients by stating that the main findings are consistent among the three surveys that have been conducted in the United States and in India over a fifteen-year period. The central tendencies of the data support the after-life hypothesis as it is formulated in the model we outlined briefly earlier in this paper.

References

Barrett, W.F. 1926. *Death-Bed Visions*. London: Methuen.

Garfield, C. 1975. "Consciousness Alteration and Fear of Death." *Journal of Transpersonal Psychology* 7:147-75.

Greeley, A.M. 1975. *Sociology of the Paranormal: A Reconnaissance*. Beverly Hills, Calif.: Sage Publications.

Hart, H. 1956. "Six Theories about Apparitions." *Proceedings of the Society for Psychical Research* 50:153-239.

Hart, H. 1951. *The Enigma of Survival*. Springfield, Ill.: Charles C Thomas.

Hyslop, J.H. 1908. *Psychical Research and the Resurrection.* Boston: Small, Maynard.

Kübler-Ross, E. 1976. Personal communication.

Moody, R.A., Jr. 1975. *Life After Life.* Atlanta: Mockingbird Books.

Murphy, G. 1961. *Challenge of Psychical Research.* New York: Harper and Row.

Myers, F.W.H. 1903. *Human Personality and Its Survival of Bodily Death,* 2 vols. London: Longmans, Green.

Noyes, R., Jr. 1972. "The Experience of Dying." *Psychiatry* 35:174:83.

Noyes, R., Jr., and R. Kletti. 1972. "The Experience of Dying from Falls." *Omega* 3:45-52.

Noyes, R., Jr., and R. Kletti. 1976. "Depersonalization in the Face of Life-Threatening Danger: A Description." *Psychiatry:* 39:19-27.

Osis, K. 1961. *Deathbed Observations by Physicians and Nurses.* New York: Parapsychology Foundation.

Rees, W.D. 1971. "The Hallucinations of Widows." *British Medical Journal* 4:37-41.

Roll, W.G. 1974. "Survival Research: Problems and Possibilities." *Theta* 39-40, 1-13.

Sidgwick, E.M. (Mrs. H.). 1923. "Phantasms of the Living." *Proceedings of the Society for Psychical Research* 33:23-429.

Sidgwick, H., and Committee. 1894. "Report on the Census of Hallucinations." *Proceedings of the Society for Psychical Research* 10:25-422.

Siegel, R.K., and L.J. West (Eds.). 1975. *Hallucinations: Behavior, Experience and Theory.* New York: Wiley.

Stevenson, I. 1974a. *Twenty Cases Suggestive of Reincarnation.* 2nd ed. rev. Charlottesville: University Press of Virginia.

Stevenson, I. 1974b. *Xenoglossy: A Review and Report of a Case.* Charlottesville: University Press of Virginia.

Stevenson, I. 1975. *Cases of the Reincarnation Type. Vol. I. Ten Cases in India.* Charlottesville: University Press of Virginia.

Tyrrell, G.N.M. 1953. *Apparitions.* London: Duckworth.

West, D.J. 1948. "A Mass Observation Questionnaire on Hallucinations." *Journal of the Society for Psychical Research* 34:187-96.

West, L.J. (Ed.). 1962. *Hallucinations.* New York: Grune and Stratton.

6

The Experience of Dying

Raymond A. Moody, Jr.

DESPITE THE WIDE VARIATION IN THE circumstances surrounding close calls with death and in the types of persons undergoing them, it remains true that there is a striking similarity among the accounts of the experiences themselves. In fact, the similarities among various reports are so great that one can easily pick out about fifteen separate elements which recur again and again in the mass of narratives that I have collected. On the basis of these points of likeness, let me now construct a brief, theoretically "ideal" or "complete" experience which embodies all of the common elements, in the order in which it is typical for them to occur.

A man is dying and, as he reaches the point of greatest physical distress, he hears himself pronounced dead by his doctor. He begins to hear an uncomfortable noise, a loud ringing or buzzing, and at the same time feels himself moving very rapidly through a long dark tunnel. After this, he suddenly finds himself outside of his own physical body, but still in the immediate physical environment, and he sees his own body from a distance, as though he is a spectator. He watches the resuscitation attempt from this unusual vantage point and is in a state of emotional upheaval.

After a while, he collects himself and becomes more accustomed to his odd condition. He notices that he still has a "body," but one of a very different nature and with very different powers from the

Revised by the compiler from *Life after Life* by Raymond A. Moody, Jr. (Covington, Georgia: Mockingbird Books, 1975), pp. 19-107. Reprinted by permission of the author and publisher. Copyright © 1975 by Raymond A. Moody, Jr.

physical body he has left behind. Soon other things begin to happen. Others come to meet and help him. He glimpses the spirits of relatives and friends who have already died, and a loving, warm spirit of a kind he has never encountered before—a being of light—appears before him. This being asks him a question, nonverbally, to make him evaluate his life and helps him along by showing him a panoramic, instantaneous playback of the major events of his life. At some point he finds himself approaching some sort of barrier or border, apparently representing the limit between earthly life and the next life. Yet, he finds that he must go back to the earth, that the time for his death has not yet come. At this point he resists, for by now he is taken up with his experiences in the afterlife and does not want to return. He is overwhelmed by intense feelings of joy, love, and peace. Despite his attitude, though, he somehow reunites with his physical body and lives.

Later he tries to tell others, but he has trouble doing so. In the first place, he can find no human words adequate to describe these unearthly episodes. He also finds that others scoff, so he stops telling other people. Still, the experience affects his life profoundly, especially his views about death and its relationship to life.

It is important to bear in mind that the above narrative is not meant to be a representation of any one person's experience; rather, it is a "model," a composite of the common elements found in very many stories. I introduce it here only to give a preliminary, general idea of what a person who is dying may experience. Since it is an abstraction rather than an actual account, in the present chapter I will discuss in detail each common element.

Before doing that, however, a few facts need to be set out in order to put the remainder of my exposition of the experience of dying into the proper framework.

1. Despite the striking similarities among various accounts, no two of them are precisely identical (though a few come remarkably close to it).

2. I have found no one person who reports every single component of the composite experience. Very many have reported most of them (that is, eight or more of the fifteen or so) and a few have reported up to twelve.

3. There is no one element of the composite experience which every single person has reported to me, which crops up in every narrative. Nonetheless, a few of these elements come fairly close to being universal.

4. There is not one component of my abstract model which has appeared in only one account. Each element has shown up in many separate stories.

5. The order in which a dying person goes through the various stages briefly delineated above may vary from that given in my "theoretical model." To give one example, various persons have reported seeing the "being of light" before, or at the same time, they left their physical bodies, and not as in the "model," some time afterward. However, the order in which the stages occur in the model is a very typical order, and wide variations are unusual.

6. How far into the hypothetical complete experience a dying person gets seems to depend on whether or not the person actually underwent an apparent clinical death, and if so, on how long he was in this state. In general, persons who were "dead" seem to report more florid, complete experiences than those who only came close to death, and those who were "dead" for a longer period go deeper than those who were "dead" for a shorter time.

7. I have talked to a few people who were pronounced dead, resuscitated, and came back reporting none of these common elements. Indeed, they say that they don't remember anything at all about their "deaths." Interestingly, I have talked with several persons who were actually adjudged clinically dead on separate occasions years apart, and reported experiencing nothing on one of the occasions, but having had quite involved experiences on the other.

8. It must be emphasized that I am writing primarily about reports, accounts, or narratives, which other persons have given to me verbally during interviews. Thus, when I remark that a given element of the abstract, "complete" experience does not occur in a given account, I do not mean necessarily to imply that it did not happen to the person involved. I only mean that this person did not tell me that it did occur, or that it does not definitely come out in his account that he experienced it. Within this framework, then, let us look at some of the common stages and events of the experiences of dying.

INEFFABILITY

The general understanding we have of language depends upon the existence of a broad community of common experience in which almost all of us participate. This fact creates an important difficulty which complicated all of the discussion which is to follow. The events which those who have come near death have lived through lie outside our community of experience, so one might well expect that they would have some linguistic difficulties in expressing what happened to them. In fact, this is precisely the case. The persons involved uniformly characterize their experiences as ineffable, that is, "inexpressible."

Many people have made remarks to the effect that, "There are just no words to express what I am trying to say," or "They just don't make adjectives and superlatives to describe this."

HEARING THE NEWS

Numerous people have told of hearing their doctors or other spectators in effect pronounce them dead. For example, one doctor told me,

> A woman patient of mine had a cardiac arrest just before another surgeon and I were to operate on her. I was right there, and I saw her pupils dilate. We tried for some time to resuscitate her, but weren't having any success, so I thought she was gone. I told the other doctor who was working with me, "Let's try one more time and then we'll give up." This time, we got her heart beating, and she came around. Later I asked her what she remembered of her "death." She said she didn't remember much about it, except that she did hear me say, "Let's try one more time and then we'll give up."

FEELINGS OF PEACE AND QUIET

Many people describe extremely pleasant feelings and sensations during the early stages of their experiences. After a severe head injury, one man's vital signs were undetectable. As he says,

> At the point of injury there was a momentary flash of pain, but then all the pain vanished. I had the feeling of floating in a dark space. The day was bitterly cold, yet while I was in that blackness all I felt was warmth and the most extreme comfort I have ever experienced.... I remember thinking, "I must be dead."

THE NOISE

In many cases, various unusual auditory sensations are reported to occur at or near death. Sometimes these are extremely unpleasant. A man who "died" for twenty minutes during an abdominal operation describes "a really bad buzzing noise coming from inside my head. It made me very uncomfortable.... I'll never forget that noise." Another woman tells how as she lost consciousness she heard a "loud ringing. It could be described as a buzzing. And I was in a sort of whirling state." I have also heard this annoying sensation described as a loud click, a roaring, a banging, and as a "whistling sound, like the wind."

In other cases the auditory effects seem to take a more pleasant musical form.

A young woman who nearly died from internal bleeding associated with a blood clotting disorder says that at the moment she collapsed, "I began to hear music of some sort, a majestic, really beautiful sort of music."

THE DARK TUNNEL

Often concurrently with the occurrence of the noise, people have the sensation of being pulled very rapidly through a dark space of some kind. Many different words are used to describe this space. I have heard this space described as a cave, a well, a trough, an enclosure, a tunnel, a funnel, a vacuum, a void, a sewer, a valley, and a cylinder. Although people use different terminology here, it is clear that they are all trying to express some one idea.

OUT OF THE BODY

It is a truism that most of us, most of the time, identify ourselves with our physical bodies. We grant, of course, that we have "minds," too. But to most people our "minds" seem much more ephemeral than our bodies. The "mind," after all, might be no more than the effect of the electrical and chemical activity which takes place in the brain, which is a part of the physical body. For many people it is an impossible task even to conceive of what it would be like to exist in any other way than in the physical body to which they are accustomed.

Prior to their experiences, the persons I have interviewed were not, as a group, any different from the average person with respect to this attitude. That is why, after his rapid passage through the dark tunnel, a dying person often has such an overwhelming surprise. For, at this point he may find himself looking upon his own physical body from a point outside of it, as though he were "a spectator" or "a third person in the room" or watching figures and events "onstage in a play" or "in a movie."

As one might well imagine, some unparalleled thoughts and feelings run through the minds of persons who find themselves in this predicament. Many people find the notion of being out of their bodies so unthinkable that, even as they are experiencing it they feel conceptually quite confused about the whole thing and do not link it with death for a considerable time. They wonder what is happening to them; why can they suddenly see themselves from a distance, as though a spectator?

Emotional responses to this strange state vary widely. Most people report, at first, a desperate desire to get back into their bodies but they do not have the faintest idea about how to proceed. Others recall that they were very afraid, almost panicky. Some, however, report more positive reactions to their plight, as in this account:

> I became very seriously ill, and the doctor put me in the hospital. This one morning a solid gray mist gathered around me, and I left my body. I had a floating sensation as I felt myself get out of my body, and I looked back and I could see myself on the bed below and there was no fear. It was quiet—very peaceful and serene. I was not in the least bit upset or frightened. It was just a tranquil feeling, and it was something which I didn't dread. I felt that maybe I was dying, and I felt that if I did not get back to my body, I would be dead, gone.

Just as strikingly variable are the attitudes which different persons take to the bodies which they have left behind. It is common for a person to report feelings of concern for his body. One young woman who was a nursing student at the time of her experience expressed fear of her body being used as a cadaver.

In another case, this concern took the form of regret.

Several persons have told me of having feelings of unfamiliarity toward their bodies.

Some persons have told me that they had no particular feelings at all toward their bodies.

Despite the eeriness of the disembodied state, the situation has been thrust upon the dying person so suddenly that it may take some time before the significance of what he is experiencing dawns upon him. He may be out of his body for some time, desperately trying to sort out all the things that are happening to him and that are racing through his mind, before he realizes that he is dying, or even dead.

When this realization comes, it may arrive with powerful emotional force, and provoke startling thoughts. One woman remembers thinking, "Oh, I'm dead! How lovely!"

A man states that the thought came to him, "This must be what they call 'death.'" Even when this realization comes, it may be accompanied by bafflement and even a certain refusal to accept one's state. One man, for example, remembers reflecting upon the Biblical promise of "three score and ten" years, and protesting that he had had "just barely one score."

In one or two cases I have studied, dying persons whose souls, minds, consciousnesses (or whatever you want to label them) were released from their bodies say that they didn't feel that, after release, they were in any kind of "body" at all. They felt as though they were "pure" consciousness. One man relates that during his experience he felt as though he were "able to see everything around me—including my whole body as it lay on the bed—without occupying space," that is, as if he were a point of consciousness. A few others say that they can't really remember whether or not they were in any kind of "body" after getting out of their physical ones, because they were so taken up with the events around them.

Far and away the majority of my subjects, however, report that they did find themselves in another body upon release from the physical one. Immediately, though, we are into an area with which it is extremely difficult to deal. This "new body" is one of the two or three aspects of death experiences in which the inadequacy of human language presents the greatest obstacles. Almost everyone who has told me of this "body" has at some point become frustrated and said, "I can't describe it," or made some remark to the same effect.

Nonetheless, the accounts of this body bear a strong resemblance to one another. Thus, although different individuals use different words and draw different analogies, these varying modes of expression do seem to fall very much within the same arena. The various reports are also in very decided agreement about the general properties and characteristics of the new body. So, to adopt a term for it which will sum up its properties fairly well, and which has been used by a couple of my subjects, I shall henceforth call it the "spiritual body."

Dying persons are likely first to become aware of their spiritual bodies in the guise of their limitations. They find, when out of their physical bodies, that although they may try desperately to tell others of their plight, no one seems to hear them.

To complicate the fact that he is apparently inaudible to people around him, the person in a spiritual body soon finds that he is also invisible to others. The medical personnel or others congregating round his physical body may look straight towards where he is, in his spiritual body, without giving the slightest sign of ever seeing him. His spiritual body also lacks solidity; physical objects in the environment appear to move through it with ease, and he is unable to get a grip on any object or person he tries to touch.

Further, it is invariably reported that this spiritual body is also weightless. Most first notice this when, as in some of the excerpts given above, they find themselves floating right up to the ceiling of the room, or into the air. Many describe a "floating sensation," "a feeling of weightlessness," or a "drifting feeling" in association with their new bodies.

Normally, while in our physical bodies, we have many modes of perception which tells us where our bodies and their various parts are in space at any given moment and whether they are moving. Vision and the sense of equilibrium are important in this respect, of course, but there is another related sense. Kinesthesia is our sense of motion or tension in our tendons, joints, and muscles. We are not usually aware of the sensations coming to us through our kinesthetic sense because our perception of it has become dulled through almost constant use. I suspect, however, that if it were suddenly to be cut off, one would immediately notice its absence. And, in fact, quite a few persons have commented to me that they were aware of the lack of the physical sensations of body weight, movement, and position sense while in their spiritual bodies.

These characteristics of the spiritual body which at first seem to be limitations can, with equal validity, be looked upon as the absence of limitations. Think of it this way: A person in the spiritual body is in a privileged position in relation to the other persons around him. He can see and hear them, but they can't see or hear him. Likewise, though the doorknob seems to go through his hand when he touches it, it really doesn't matter anyway, because he soon finds that he can just *go through* the door. Travel, once one gets the hang of it, is apparently exceptionally easy in this state. Physical objects present no barrier, and movement from one place to another can be extremely rapid, almost instantaneous.

Furthermore, despite its lack of perceptibility to people in physical bodies, all who have experienced it are in agreement that the spiritual body is nonetheless *something,* impossible to describe though it may be. It is agreed that the spiritual body has a form or shape (sometimes a globular or an amorphous cloud, but also sometimes essentially the same shape as the physical body) and even parts (projections or surfaces analogous to arms, legs, a head, etc.). Even when its shape is reported as being generally roundish in configuration, it is often said to have ends, a definite top and bottom, and even the "parts" just mentioned.

I have heard this new body described in many different terms, but one may readily see that much the same idea is being formulated in each case. Words and phrases which have been used by various subjects include a mist, a cloud, smoke-like, a vapor, transparent, a cloud of colors, wispy, an energy pattern, and others which express similar meanings.

Finally, almost everyone remarks upon the *timelessness* of this out-of-body state. Many say that although they must describe their interlude in the spiritual body in temporal terms (since human language is temporal), time was not really an element of their experience as it is in physical life.

In their accounts, others have briefly mentioned the likeness of shape between their physical bodies and their new ones. One woman told me that while out of her body, "I still felt an entire body form, legs, arms, everything—even while I was weightless." A lady who watched the resuscitation attempt on her body from a point just below the ceiling says, "I was still in a body. I was stretched out and looking down. I moved my legs and noticed that one of them felt warmer than the other one."

Just as movement is unimpeded in this spiritual state, so, some recall, is thought. Over and over, I have been told that once they became accustomed to their new situation, people undergoing this experience began to think more lucidly and rapidly than in physical existence.

Perception in the new body is both like and unlike perception in the physical body. In some ways, the spiritual form is more limited. As we saw, kinesthesia, as such, is absent. In a couple of instances, persons have reported that they had no sensation of temperature, while in most cases feelings of comfortable "warmth" are reported. No one among all of my cases has reported any odors or tastes while out of their physical bodies.

On the other hand, senses which correspond to the physical senses of vision and of hearing are very definitely intact in the spiritual body, and seem actually heightened and more perfect than they are in physical life. One man says that while he was "dead" his vision seemed incredibly more powerful and, in his words, "I just can't understand how I could see so far." A woman who recalled this experience notes, "It seemed as if this spiritual sense had no limitations, as if I could look anywhere and everywhere."

"Hearing" in the spiritual state can apparently be called so only by analogy, and most say that they do not really hear physical voices or sounds. Rather, they seem to pick up the thoughts of persons around them, and, as we shall see later, this same kind of direct transfer of thoughts can play an important role in the late stages of death experiences.

Finally, on the basis of one unique and very interesting report, it would appear that even severe damage to the physical body in no way adversely affects the spiritual one. In this case, a man lost the better part of his leg in the accident that resulted in his clinical death. He knew this, because he saw his damaged body clearly, from a distance, as the doctor worked on it. Yet, while he was out of his body,

> I could feel my body, and it was whole. I know that. I felt whole, and I felt that all of me was there, though it wasn't.

In this disembodied state, then, a person is cut off from others. He can see other people and understand their thoughts completely, but they are able neither to see nor to hear him. Communication with other human beings is effectively cut off, even through the sense of touch, since his spiritual body lacks solidity. Thus, it is not surprising that after a time in this state profound feelings of isolation and loneliness set in. As one man put it, he could see everything around him in the hospital—all the doctors, nurses, and other personnel going about their tasks. Yet, he could not communicate with them in any way, so "I was desperately alone."

The dying person's feelings of loneliness are soon dispelled, however, as he gets deeper into his near-death experience. For, at some point, others come to him to give him aid in the transition he is undergoing. These may take the form of other spirits, often those of deceased relatives or friends the individual had known while he was alive. In a greater number of instances, among those I interviewed, a spiritual being of a much different character appears. In the next few sections we will look at such encounters.

MEETING OTHERS

Quite a few have told me that at some point while they were dying—sometimes early in the experience, sometimes only after other events had taken place—they became aware of the presence of other spiritual beings in their vicinity, beings who apparently were there to ease them through their transition into death, or, in two cases, to tell them that their time to die had not yet come and that they must return to their physical bodies.

In other cases, the spirits people encounter are not persons whom they knew in physical life. One woman told of seeing during her out-of-body experience not only her own transparent spiritual body but also another one, that of another person who had died very recently. She did not know who this person was, but made the very interesting remark that "I did not see this person, this spirit, as having any particular *age,* at all. I didn't even have any sense of time myself."

In a very few instances, people have come to believe that the beings they encountered were their "guardian spirits." One man was told by such a spirit that, "I have helped you through this stage of your existence, but now I am going to turn you over to others." A woman told me that as she was leaving her body she detected the presence of two other spiritual beings there, and that they identified themselves as her "spiritual helpers."

In two very similar cases, persons told me of hearing a voice which told them that they were not dead yet, but that they must go back.

Finally, the spiritual beings may take a somewhat more amorphous form.

THE BEING OF LIGHT

What is perhaps the most incredible common element in the accounts I have studied, and is certainly the element which has the most profound effect upon the individual, is the encounter with a very bright light. Typically, at its first appearance this light is dim, but it rapidly gets brighter until it reaches an unearthly brilliance. Yet, even though this light (usually said to be white or "clear") is of an indescribable brilliance, many make the specific point that it does not in any way hurt their eyes, or dazzle them, or keep them from seeing other things around them (perhaps because at this point they don't have physical "eyes" to be dazzled).

Despite the light's unusual manifestation, however, not one person has expressed any doubt whatsoever that it was a being, a being of light. Not only that, it is a personal being. It has a very definite personality. The love and the warmth which emanate from this being to the dying person are utterly beyond words, and he feels completely surrounded by it and taken up in it, completely at ease and accepted in the presence of this being. He senses an irresistible magnetic attraction to this light. He is ineluctably drawn to it.

Interestingly, while the above description of the being of light is utterly invariable, the identification of the being varies from individual to individual and seems to be largely a function of the religious background, training, or beliefs of the person involved. Thus, most of those who are Christians in training or belief identify the light as Christ and sometimes draw biblical parallels in support of their interpretation. A Jewish man and woman identified the light as an "angel." It was clear, though, in both cases, that the subjects did not mean to imply that the being had wings, played a harp, or even had a human shape or appearance. There was only the light. What each was trying to get across was that the being acted as an emissary, or a guide. A man who had had no religious beliefs or training at all prior to his experience simply identified what he saw as "a being of light." The same label was used by one lady of the Christian faith, who apparently did not feel any compulsion at all to call the light "Christ."

Shortly after its appearance, the being begins to communicate with the person who is passing over. Notably, this communication is of the same direct kind which we encountered earlier in the description of how a person in the spiritual body may "pick up the thoughts" of those around him. For, here again, people claim that they did not hear any physical voice or sounds coming from the being, nor did they respond to the being through audible sounds. Rather, it is reported that direct, unimpeded transfer of thoughts takes place, and in such a clear way that there is no possibility whatsoever either of misunderstanding or of lying to the light.

Furthermore, this unimpeded exchange does not even take place in the native language of the person. Yet, he understands perfectly and is instantaneously aware. He cannot even translate the thoughts and exchanges which took place while he was near death into the human language which he must speak now, after his resuscitation.

The next step of the experience clearly illustrates the difficulty of translating from this unspoken language. The being almost immediately directs a certain thought to the person into whose presence it has come so dramatically. Usually the persons with whom I have talked try to formulate the thought into a question. Among the translations I have heard are: "Are you prepared to die?" "Are you ready to die?" "What have you done with your life to show me?" and "What have you done with your life that is sufficient?" The first two formulations which stress "preparation," might at first seem to have a different sense from the second pair, which emphasize "accomplishment."

This question, ultimate and profound as it may be in its emotional impact is not at all asked in condemnation. The being, all seem to agree, does not direct the question to them to accuse or to threaten them, for they still feel the total love and acceptance coming from the light, no matter what their answer may be. Rather, the point of the question seems to be to make them think about their lives, to draw them out. It is, if you will, a Socratic question, one asked not to acquire information but to help the person who is being asked to proceed along the path to the truth by himself.

THE REVIEW

The initial appearance of the being of light and his probing, non-verbal questions are the prelude to a moment of startling intensity during which the being presents to the person a panoramic review of his life. It is often obvious that the being can see the individual's whole life displayed and that he doesn't himself need information. His only intention is to provoke reflection.

This review can only be described in terms of memory, since that is the closest familiar phenomenon to it, but it has characteristics which set it apart from any normal type of remembering. First of all, it is extraordinarily rapid. The memories, when they are described in temporal terms, are said to follow one another swiftly, in chronological order. Others recall no awareness of temporal order at all. The remembrance was instantaneous; everything appeared at once, and they could take it all in with one mental glance. However it is expressed, all seem in agreement that the experience was over in an instant of earthly time.

Yet, despite its rapidity, my informants agree that the review, almost always described as a display of visual imagery, is incredibly vivid and real. In some cases, the images are reported to be in vibrant color, three dimensional, and even moving. And even if they are flickering rapidly by, each image is perceived and recognized. Even the emotions and feelings associated with the images may be re-experienced as one is viewing them.

Some of those I interviewed claim that, while they cannot adequately explain it, everything they had ever done was there in this review—from the most insignificant to the most meaningful. Others explain that what they saw were mainly the highlights of their lives. Some have stated to me that even for a period of time following their experience of the review they could recall the events of their lives in incredible detail.

Some people characterize this as an educational effort on the part of the being of light. As they witness the display, the being seems to stress the importance of two things in life: Learning to love other people and acquiring knowledge.

It must also be pointed out that reports exist in which the review is experienced even though the being of light does not appear. As a rule, in experiences in which the being does apparently "direct" it, the review is a more overwhelming experience. Nonetheless, it is usually characterized as quite vivid and rapid, and as accurate, regardless of whether or not the being of light appears, and regardless of whether it occurs in the course of an actual "death" or only during a close brush with death.

The Border or Limit

In a few instances, persons have described to me how during their near-death experience they seemed to be approaching what might be called a border or a limit of some kind. This has taken the form, in various accounts, of a body of water, a gray mist, a door, a fence across a field, or simply a line. Though this is highly speculative, one could raise the question of whether there might not be some one basic experience or idea at the root of all of them. If this is true, then the different versions would merely represent varying individual ways of interpreting, wording, or remembering the root experience. Let us look at an account in which the idea of a border or limit plays a prominent role.

I had a heart attack, and I found myself in a black void, and I knew I had left my physical body behind. I knew I was dying, and I thought, "God, I did the best I knew how at the time I did it. Please help me." Immediately, I was moved out of that blackness, through a pale gray, and I just went on, gliding and moving swiftly, and in front of me, in the distance, I could see a gray mist, and I was rushing toward it. It seemed that I just couldn't get to it fast enough to satisfy me, and as I got closer to it I could see through it. Beyond the mist, I could see people, and their forms were just like they are on the earth, and I could also see something which one could take to be buildings. The whole thing was permeated with the most gorgeous light—a living, golden yellow glow, a pale color, not like the harsh gold color we know on earth.

As I approached more closely, I felt certain that I was going through that mist. It was such a wonderful, joyous feeling; there are just no words in human language to describe it. Yet, it wasn't my time to go through the mist, because instantly from the other side appeared my Uncle Carl, who had died many years earlier. He blocked my path, saying, "Go back. Your work on earth has not been completed. Go back now." I didn't want to go back, but I had no choice, and immediately I was back in my body. I felt that horrible pain in my chest, and I heard my little boy crying, "God, bring my mommy back to me."

COMING BACK

Obviously, all the persons with whom I have talked had to "come back" at some point in their experience. Usually, though, an interesting change in their attitude had taken place by this time. Remember that the most common feelings reported in the first few moments following death are a desperate desire to get back into the body and an intense regret over one's demise. However, once the dying person reaches a certain depth in his experience, he does not want to come back, and he may even resist the return to the body. This is especially the case for those who have gotten so far as to encounter the being of light. As one man put it, most emphatically, "I *never* wanted to leave the presence of this being."

Exceptions to this generalization are often only apparent, not real. Several women who were mothers of young children at the time of their experience have told me that, while for *themselves* they would have preferred to stay where they were, they felt an obligation to try to go back and to raise their children.

In several other cases, persons have told me that, though they were comfortable and secure in their new disembodied existence and were even enjoying it, they felt happy to be able to return to physical life since they had left some important task undone. In a few cases, this has taken the form of a desire to complete an unfinished education.

The accounts I have collected present an extremely varied picture when it comes to the question of the mode of return to physical life and of why the return took place. Most say simply that they do not know how or why they returned, or that they can only make guesses. A few very definitely feel that their own decisions to get back to the body and to return to earthly life were the operative factors.

Others feel that they were in effect *allowed* to live by "God," or by the being of light, either in response to their own request to be allowed to live (usually because the request was made unselfishly) or because God or the being apparently had some mission in mind for them to fulfill.

As one man remembers:

I say God surely was good to me, because I was dead, and he let the doctors bring me back, for a purpose. The purpose was to help my wife, I think, because she had a drinking problem, and I know that she just couldn't have made it without me. She is better now, though, and I really think it had a lot to do with what I went through.

In a few instances, persons have expressed the feeling that the love or prayers of others have in effect pulled them back from death regardless of their own wishes.

In quite a few instances, persons recall being drawn rapidly back through the dark tunnel through which they went during the initial moments of their experience. One man who died, for example, relates how he was propelled forward through a dark valley. He felt he was approaching the end of the tunnel, yet just at that moment he heard his name called from behind. He then was drawn backwards through the same space.

Few experience the actual re-entry into their physical bodies. Most report that they simply felt that at the end of their experience they "went to sleep" or lapsed into unconsciousness, later to awaken in their physical bodies.

On the other hand, some remember being drawn speedily back towards their physical bodies, often with a jerk, at the end of their experiences.

In the very few accounts in which the event is recalled in some detail, re-entry is said to occur "through the head."

Typically, the moods and feelings which were associated with the experience linger on for some time after the actual medical crisis has been resolved.

TELLING OTHERS

It must be emphasized that a person who has been through an experience of this type has no doubt whatsoever as to its reality and its importance. Interviews which I have done are usually sprinkled with remarks to precisely that effect.

Such remarks come from persons who are very capable of distinguishing dream and fantasy from reality. The people I have interviewed are functional, well-balanced personalities. Yet, they do not tell their experiences as they would dreams, but rather as real events which actually happened to them.

Despite their own certainty of the reality and importance of what has happened to them, they realize that our contemporary society is just not the sort of environment in which reports of this nature would be received with sympathy and understanding. Indeed, many have remarked that they realized from the very beginning that others would think they were mentally unstable if they were to relate their experiences. So, they have resolved to remain silent on the subject or else to reveal their experiences only to some very close relative.

Others tried at first to tell someone else, but were rebuffed, so they resolved from then on to remain silent.

Interestingly enough, in only one of the cases I have studied did a physician reveal any familiarity at all with near-death experiences or express any sympathy with them.

Considering the skepticism and lack of understanding that greet the attempt of a person to discuss his near-death experience, it is not surprising that almost everyone in this situation comes to feel that he is unique, that no one else has ever undergone what he has. For example, one man told me, "I have been somewhere nobody else has ever been."

It has often happened that when, after first interviewing someone in detail about his own experience, I have proceeded to tell him that others have reported exactly the same events and perceptions, he has expressed profound feelings of relief.

There is yet another reason why some are reticent to relate their experiences to others. They feel that the experience is so indescribable, so far beyond human language and human modes of perception and existence, that it is fruitless even to try.

EFFECTS ON LIVES

For the reasons just explained, no one in my experience has built himself a portable lectern and gone out to preach about his experience on a full-time basis. No one has seen fit to proselytize, to try to convince others of the realities he experienced. Indeed, I have found that the difficulty is quite the reverse: People are naturally very reticent to tell others about what happened to them.

The effects which their experiences have had on their lives seem to have taken subtler, quieter forms. Many have told me that they felt that their lives were broadened and deepened by their experience, that because of it they became more reflective and more concerned with ultimate philosophical issues.

Others report a changed attitude or approach towards the physical life to which they have returned. One woman, for instance, says quite simply that "it made life much more precious to me."

A few have mentioned that what they underwent changed their concepts of the mind and of the relative importance of the physical body as against the mind.

In a very small number of cases, persons have told me that after their experiences they seemed to acquire or to notice faculties of intuition bordering on the psychic.

There is a remarkable agreement in the "lessons," as it were, which have been brought back from these close encounters with death. Almost everyone has stressed the importance in this life of trying to cultivate love for others, a love of a unique and profound kind. One man who met the being of light felt totally loved and accepted, even while his whole life was displayed in a panorama for the being to see. He felt that the "question" that the being was asking him was whether he was able to love others in the same way. He now feels that it is his commission while on earth to try to learn to be able to do so.

In addition, many others have emphasized the importance of seeking knowledge. During their experiences, it was intimated to them that the acquisition of knowledge continues even in the afterlife. One woman, for example, has taken advantage of every educational opportunity she has had since her "death" experience. Another man offers the advice, "No matter how old you are, don't stop learning. For this is a process, I gather, that goes on for eternity."

No one that I interviewed has reported coming out of this experience feeling morally "purified" or perfected. No one with whom I have talked in any way evinces a "holier-than-thou" attitude. In fact, most have specifically brought up the point that they feel that they are still trying, still searching. Their vision left them with new goals, new moral principles, and a renewed determination to try to live in accordance with them, but with no feelings of instantaneous salvation or of moral infallibility.

NEW VIEWS OF DEATH

As one might reasonably expect, this experience has a profound effect upon one's attitude towards physical death, especially for those who had not previously expected that anything took place after death. In some form or another, almost every person has expressed to me the thought that he is no longer afraid of death. This requires clarification, though. In the first place, certain modes of death are obviously undesirable, and secondly, none of these persons are actively seeking death. They all feel that they have tasks to do as long as they are physically alive and would agree with the words of a man who told me, "I've got quite a lot of changing to do before I leave here." Likewise, all would disavow suicide as a means by which to return to the realms they glimpsed during their experiences. It is just that now the state of death itself is no longer forbidding to them.

The reason why death is no longer frightening, is that after his experience a person no longer entertains any doubts about his survival of bodily death. It is no longer merely an abstract possibility to him, but a fact of his experience.

Persons who have "died" choose analogies which portray death as a transition from one state to another, or as an entry into a higher state of consciousness or of being. One woman, whose deceased relatives were there to greet her at her death, compared death to a "homecoming." Others have likened it to other psychologically positive states, for example, to awakening, to graduating, and to escape from jail.

Even those who previously had some traditional conviction about the nature of the afterlife world seem to have moved away from it to some degree following their own brushes with death. In fact, in all the reports I have gathered, not one person has painted the mythological picture of what lies hereafter. No one has described the cartoonist's heaven of pearly gates, golden streets, and winged, harp-playing angels, nor a hell of flames and demons with pitchforks.

So, in most cases, the reward-punishment model of the afterlife is abandoned and disavowed, even by many who had been accustomed to thinking in those terms. They found, much to their amazement, that even when their most apparently awful and sinful deeds were made manifest before the being of light, the being responded not with anger and rage, but rather only with understanding, and even with humor. As one woman went through the review of her life with this being, she saw some scenes in which she had failed to show love and had shown selfishness. Yet, she says, "His attitude when we came to these scenes was just that I had been learning, even then." In place of this old model, many seemed to have returned with a new model and a new understanding of the world beyond—a vision which features not unilateral judgement, but rather cooperative development towards the ultimate end of self-realization. According to these new views, development of the soul, especially in the spiritual faculties of love and knowledge, does not stop upon death. Rather, it continues on the other side, perhaps eternally, but certainly for a period of time and to a depth which can only be glimpsed, while we are still in physical bodies, "through a glass, darkly."

CORROBORATION

The question naturally arises whether any evidence of the reality of near-death experiences might be acquired independently of the descriptions of the experiences themselves. Many persons report being out of their bodies for extended periods and witnessing many events in the physical world during the interlude. Can any of these reports be checked out with other witnesses who were known to be present, or with later confirming events, and thus be corroborated?

In quite a few instances, the somewhat surprising answer to this question is "yes." Furthermore, the descriptions of events witnessed while out of the body tend to check out fairly well. Several doctors have told me, for example, that they are utterly baffled about how patients with no medical knowledge could describe in such detail and so correctly the procedure used in resuscitation attempts, even though these events took place while the doctors knew the patients involved to be "dead."

In several cases, persons have related to me how they amazed their doctors or others with reports of events they had witnessed while out of the body. While she was dying, for example, one girl went out of her body and into another room in the hospital where she found her older sister crying and saying, "Oh, Kathy, please don't die, please don't die." The older sister was quite baffled when later Kathy told her exactly where she had been and what she had been saying during this time.

Finally, in a few cases, I have been able to get the independent testimony of others about corroborating events. In assessing the evidential value of such independent reports, however, several complicating factors arise. First, in most of the cases the corroborating event itself is attested to only by the dying person himself and by at most a couple of close friends and acquaintances. Second, even in the exceptionally dramatic, well-attested instances I have collected, I have promised not to reveal actual names. Even if I could, though, I do not think that such corroborating stories collected after the fact would constitute *proof.*

7

Frequency and Stages of the Prototypic Near-Death Experience[1]

Kenneth Ring

BEGINNING IN MAY 1977, my research staff and I spent thirteen months tracking down and interviewing persons who had come close to death. In some cases, these were persons who appeared to suffer "clinical" death, where there is no heartbeat or respiration; in most cases, however, the individuals we talked with had undergone a near-death crisis which stopped short of "clinical" death.

I was led to undertake this research as a direct result of reading Dr. Raymond Moody's first book, *Life After Life* (1975). As the readers of this volume will know, Moody delineates a common pattern of near-death experience elements. In doing so, Moody stresses that his is an idealized conceptualization and represents a *composite* experience, not an actual one. He further comments that different persons in his sample approximated this ideal, but no one person reported every single feature of this prototypic account. Since Moody's formulation was the starting point of my own research, it perhaps should be quoted again here.

A man is dying and, as he reaches the point of greatest physical distress, he hears himself pronounced dead by his doctor. He begins to hear an uncomfortable noise, a loud ringing or buzzing, and at the same time feels himself moving very rapidly through a long tunnel. After this, he suddenly finds himself outside his own physical body, but still in the same immediate physical environment, and sees his own body from a distance as though he is a spectator. He watches the resuscitation attempt from this vantage point and is in a state of emotional upheaval....

After a while, he collects himself and becomes more accustomed to his odd condition. He notices that he still has a "body," but one of a very different nature and with very different powers from the physical body he has left behind. Some other things begin to happen. Others come to meet him and help him. He glimpses the spirits of relatives and friends who have already died, and a loving, warm spirit of a kind he has never encountered before—a being of light—appears before him. This being asks him a question, nonverbally, to make him evaluate his life and helps him along by showing him a panoramic, instantaneous playback of the major events of his life. At some point, he finds himself approaching some sort of a barrier or border, apparently representing the limit between earthly life and the next life. Yet, he finds that he must go back to the earth, that the time for his death has not yet come. At this point he resists, for by now he is taken up with his experiences in the afterlife and does not want to return. He is overwhelmed by intense feelings of joy, love, and peace. Despite his attitude, though, he somehow reunites with his physical body and lives....

Later he tries to tell others, but he has trouble doing so. In the first place, he can find no human words to describe these unearthly episodes. He also finds that others scoff, so he stops telling other people. Still, the experience affects his life profoundly, especially his views about death and its relationship to life. [Moody, 1975, p. 23-24]

Although this description is based on some one hundred fifty cases, Moody's research methodology and his failure to provide any statistical data obviously leave the critical reader with many questions still unanswered. For example, how commonly does the basic near-death pattern occur? (In his book, Moody gives the reader only the positive instances, only the "hits," as it were.) Are some elements of the pattern more common than others? How rich or detailed is the modal near-death experience? Does it make a difference how one almost dies? (Thus, do failed suicides undergo the same kind of near-death experience as individuals who suffer a cardiac arrest?) What role does prior religiosity play in shaping those experiences? Can the changes that allegedly follow from these experiences be documented systematically and quantitatively? Our study was designed to provide at least some preliminary answers to these questions.

In this article, I shall confine myself to two issues: (1) the frequency with which Moody-type experiences[2] occur in a sample of near-death survivors and (2) the manner in which this experience tends to unfold.[3] In relation to this second issue, I shall present a conceptualization of the stages of the core experience and furnish data on the relative frequency of each stage. In this way, it will be possible, I believe, to achieve a more adequate understanding of the experience of dying.

METHOD

Our study systematically compared the experiences of 102 persons who had come close to death in one of three ways: 52 had nearly died from illness; 26 had been involved in a serious accident; and 24 had made a serious suicide attempt. The majority of our respondents were obtained through a reference system set up in several hospitals in Hartford, Connecticut. Additional respondents were obtained from other sources including newspaper advertisements. In conducting this research, we were careful throughout to phrase our appeals for respondents in terms simply of their having come close to death. Having had an "experience" of some kind was not, then, a criterion of respondent selection. Thirty-six percent of our respondents were interviewed within a year of their near-death episodes; an additional 22 percent were interviewed within two years of their episode. I myself interviewed 74 of our 102 respondents; the remainder of the interviews were conducted by several graduate students working with me on the project.

Our method of data collection involved the use of a structured interview schedule. The interview itself was composed of five distinct information-gathering segments which occurred in the following order:

1. Demographic information
2. A free narrative of the near-death episode
3. A series of probing questions designed to determine the presence/absence of the various components of the core experience as delineated by Moody
4. Aftereffects
5. Pre- and post-incident comparison of religious beliefs and attitudes.

Prior to the interview, the respondent was assured of both anonymity and confidentiality. Since the interview was to be tape-recorded, appropriate justification was given for this procedure. In order not to bias the respondent's comments, most questions about the study and its underlying purposes were deferred until the end of the interview, at which time all queries were answered. Before the interviewer left, he/she left a card indicating where he/she could be reached. All interested respondents were also promised and sent a report of our findings.

Most of the interviews took between one-half and one hour to complete; none took longer than one-and-a-half hours. Most of the interviews were conducted in the respondent's home. Some took place in hospitals (usually a private room was available) and a few were held in my office or home.

Some basic demographic information on our sample is presented in Table 1. Although, for the most part, frequency data are given in Table 1, the frequencies are nearly equal to percentages since the total number of interviewees was 102. For legal reasons, no one under eighteen was interviewed. From an inspection of Table 1, it will be seen that, with the exception of youth and race, our sample of near-death survivors represents a considerable range of demographic diversity.

RESULTS: FREQUENCY OF THE CORE EXPERIENCE

In *Reflections on Life After Life* Moody (1977, pp. 88-89), in discussing what I have called the core experience, predicts that "any investigator who enters into this type of study sympathetically and diligently will find that there is ample case material."

How warranted is this assertion? In fact, just how frequent is the core experience pattern as described by Moody?

To answer this question, I constructed a near-death experience index which is essentially a weighted measure of the depth of the experience. In effect, the higher the index, the greater the number of Moody-type elements in the account. Scores on this index, which I call the Weighted Core Experience Index (WCEI) can range from a theoretical low of 0 (indicating the absence of any Moody-type experience) to 29 (representing the deepest Moody-type experience).

In using the WCEI for the purpose of classification, certain arbitrary (but, in my judgment, reasonable) cutoff points were assigned. If an individual's score was less than 6, he or she was adjudged not to have had "enough" of an experience to qualify as a "core experiencer." This doubtless eliminates some individuals who

TABLE 1

Demographic Data on Interviewees

Total interviewed	102
Sex	
Male	45
Female	57
Race	
White	97
Black	5
Marital Status	
Married	47
Single	32
Divorced/Separated	16
Widowed	7
Religious Denomination	
Catholic	37
Protestant	34
None	21
Other	3
Agnostic/Atheist	7
Education	
College Graduate	11
Some College/College Student	34
High School Graduate	39
Some High School	10
Grade School Only	8
Age Range	18-84
Mean age at interview	43.91
Mean age of near-death incident	37.81

might have been included by Moody (indeed, it was my impression that this index failed to include some interviewees who probably did experience some aspects of the Moody pattern), but it seems to me better to err on the side of under inclusion. Individuals scoring between 6 and 9 on the WCEI will be designated "moderate experiencers" and individuals with scores in excess of 10 will be referred to as "deep experiencers."

In evaluating our near-death accounts in this way, I found Moody's assertion upheld concerning the abundance of these experiences. Altogether forty-nine of our cases, or 48 percent of our entire sample, recounted experiences which conform in an obvious way to Moody's core experience pattern. Our evidence on this point, then, is in total accord with Moody's findings and those of other near-death researchers.

In terms of the tripartite classification scheme mentioned above, twenty-seven persons (26 percent) were deep experiencers, twenty-two (22 percent) were moderate experiencers, and the remaining fifty-three (52 percent) were nonexperiencers. Scores on the WCEI ranged from 0 to 24. There were virtually no sex differences in either frequency or depth of the core experience. The percentages were as follows:

	Men	Women
Deep experiencers	27	26
Moderate experiencers	20	23
Nonexperiencers	53	51

In interpreting our overall core experience figures of 48 percent, it is however necessary to bear certain factors in mind. First of all, our sample of cases was not selected randomly and there is evidence of a self-selection tendency across categories of respondents (e.g., accident victims were much more likely to consent to be interviewed than were attempted suicides). Second, this figure is based on a sample of near-death cases in the approximate ratio of 2:1:1 for illness, accident, and suicide-attempt victims, respectively. Finally, the source of referral needs to be taken into account. Of those respondents who were either self-referred or referred by nonmedical sources, 58 percent reported core experiences. The corresponding figure for those (n = 59) referred by medical sources was 39 percent. Even though these percentages are not significantly different, there is reason to believe that the lower estimate is the more representative figure. Despite these methodological problems, this last estimate used as a ballpark figure is perhaps fairly accurate in the light of Sabom's (1978) finding that 42 percent of his prospective patients reported core experiences.[4]

Now that we can be reasonably confident that core experiences are not rare events in conjunction with apparent imminent death, we must try to deepen our understanding of these experiences beyond the descriptive and anecdotal level which has been characteristic of most of the early work in this field. As a first step in this direction, I want next to offer a five stage conceptualization of the core experience. In conjunction with this model, we shall also be able to see just what variation exists in the frequency of the different core experience features delineated by Moody and corroborated in our work.

STAGES OF THE CORE EXPERIENCE

In our study and comparison of near-death experiences, I found that the core experience tends to unfold in a characteristic way. In general, the earlier stages of the experience, which I shall shortly describe, are more common; the later stages manifest themselves with systematically decreasing frequency. Thus, it seems that not only are some Moody categories more common than others, but also that they are meaningfully ordered in frequency.

In Figure 1, I have indicated five distinct stages of the core experience, as suggested by our data, along with their corresponding frequency. In the subsections to follow, these five categories of experience will be described more fully and amply illustrated by reference to interviews. As this discussion proceeds, it will be apparent that when these five categories are considered *in seriatim,* they will form a coherent pattern. What we will have, then, is the basic thanatomimetic narrative—the experience of (apparent) death in its developmental form.

The Affective Component: Peace and the Sense of Well-Being

The first stage, and one which is emphasized in many of our accounts, relates to the affective accompaniment of the core experience. The conscious experience of dying is heralded by a feeling of such peace and contentment that many respondents claim there is simply no way to describe it. Nevertheless some of the attempts to do so—which I shall be quoting shortly—are themselves deeply moving and compelling, even when words do ultimately fail. As can be seen from Figure 1, about 60 percent of our sample report this kind of experience. This figure includes some who never get beyond this stage and a few who do not really conform to other aspects of the Moody pattern. If we confine ourselves to just these respondents who are "core experiencers," then 35 of 49, or 71 percent, explicitly use the words "peaceful" or "calm" to characterize

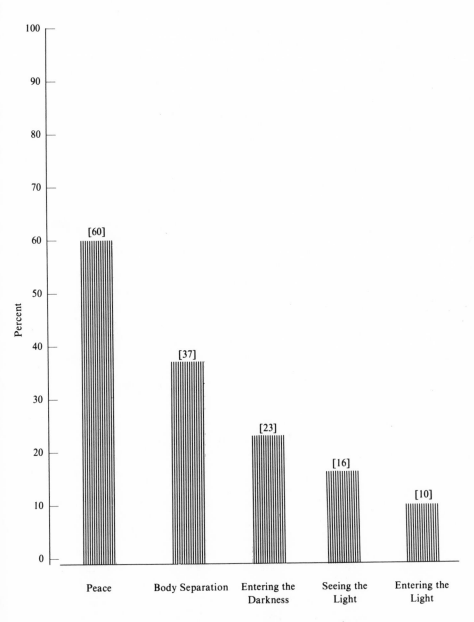

FIGURE 1.   Stages of the Near-Death Experience

the feeling-tone of their experience. Most of the others in this category, as might be inferred, use various synonyms to describe how they felt.

Before presenting a full statistical breakdown of the different aspects of the affective component accompanying the core experience, it seems necessary to provide some qualitative descriptive accounts. The illustrations given below are meant to convey something of the range of the affective response to apparent imminent death. Enough excerpts will be cited here to give, as well, a sense of "the central tendency" of these statements.

A woman who nearly died of a ruptured appendix commented:

I had a feeling of total peace. A feeling of total, total peace...it was just such a total peaceful sensation...I wasn't frightened any more.

Another woman who had a cardiac arrest stated:

[There was] nothing painful. There was nothing frightening about it. It was just something that I felt I gave myself into completely. And it felt good.... One very, very strong feeling was that if I could only make them [her doctors] understand how comfortable and how *painless* it is...how natural it is...I felt no sadness. No longing. No fear.

A woman who had attempted suicide by hurling herself into the ocean and was badly smashed by the waves against the rocks of a nearby cliff recalled:

This incredible feeling of peace [came] over me.... All of a sudden there was no pain, just peace. [Later in the interview she reflected on the sheer difficulty of describing how she felt.] I suppose it's because it's so completely unlike anything else that I've ever experienced in my life. So that I've got nothing to compare it to. A perfectly beautiful, beautiful feeling...to me, there's a definite feeling of sunlight and warmth associated with this peaceful feeling. [It should be noted that on the day this woman tried to drown herself the water temperature was 48°; she remembers feeling very cold in the ocean and was told that she shivered a great deal in the hospital afterward.] But when this feeling of peace came over me, I was warm. I felt warm, safe, happy, relaxed, just every wonderful adjective you could use.... This was perfection, this is everything anyone could possibly want and everything I could possibly want—is this, is this feeling.

In case the reader feels that these extravagant descriptions reflect a kind of female hyperbole, the following accounts from men in our sample should dispel that impression.

A race car driver commented:

> I guess the best description would be visualizing someone in a very strenuous, active sport and when they got through with it, they take a sauna and have a massage. And if you can experience that feeling of relaxation, then multiply it times one thousand, that's how you would feel. It was just super, super great.

A young man who nearly died when his fever hit 106.9° said:

> The mellowness and the passiveness that I felt in this state was just so intense... like I said before, it was a very, very strong—I can only use the word mellow feeling, passive feeling. There wasn't one bit of discontentment that I felt. I felt [pause] I can probably say the highest I've ever felt in my life.

A man who tried to hang himself recalled that:

> I felt really good. It felt, like when you wake up in the morning and you feel real good, you have a good feeling.

A man who nearly perished in a boating accident testified:

> It's tough. Use euphoric. Use orgasmic. Or use high. It was very tangible, very real. But it was doing magnificent things to me. You know, afterward I looked at that lake and I said, 'that lake made love to me.' It really did, it felt like that."

More excerpts will perhaps be redundant, but I feel that repetition here is not wasted if it serves to convey just how frequently these powerful feelings are associated with the onset of apparent death.

A 60-year-old woman who had suffered cardiac arrest observed:

> I think that probably the next thing I remember is total, peaceful, wonderful blackness. Very peaceful blackness... the only other word I might add would be softness. Just an indescribable peacefulness, absolutely indescribable. [This was] a total peacefulness, an *absolute* [said very slowly and with great emphasis] peacefulness.

A man who nearly died as a result of a motorcycle crash said, as he lay (apparently) dying in the hospital:

> I felt peaceful. I felt calm. No pain... extremely peaceful.

Next we have a woman who clearly struggled to find the words to describe the ineffable. Her comments were perhaps the most passionate of any of my respondents, but that may be because she was one of the few who attempted to articulate for me that which most others despaired of ever being able to communicate verbally. She had suffered cardiac arrest in connection with a tonsillectomy.

> The thing I could never—absolutely never forget is that absolute feeling of [pause] peace [pause] joy, or something. ... I remember the feeling. I just remember this absolute beautiful feeling. Of peace... and happy! Oh! So happy!... The *peace*... the release [pause], the fear was all gone. There was no pain. There was nothing. It was just absolutely beautiful! [said with the strongest emphasis]. I could never explain it in a million years. It was a feeling that I think everybody dreams of someday having. Reaching a point of *absolute* [said slowly and with great emphasis] peace. To me peace is the greatest word that I can express.

These excerpts should be sufficient to suggest a fairly clear impression of the feeling-tone which seems to serve both as an initial cue for the core experience and an affective background during its unfolding. A more detailed statistical picture of the range of affective reactions accompanying the core experience can be gleaned from Table 2. For purposes of comparison, I have given the percentages for both core experiencers and nonexperiencers. Even a casual inspection of Table 2 reveals several points of interest. First, the general affective response of core experiencers was extremely positive. This can be inferred from the most commonly employed adjectives to describe the experience. In fact, of the 170 feelings and emotions named by the core experiencers, only 8 (or 4.7 percent) were negative. And of these (mostly fear), most were transient in nature, occurring at the beginning of the experience or after its termination. Also, there is no clear pattern of affective responses for the nonexperiencers, even though in their case the positive qualities of peacefulness, painlessness, and the absence of fear maintain the same relative rankings. Nevertheless, despite the identical ranking of the first three characteristics, it is obvious that the percentage values are drastically lower. Even then, because of the conservative nature of our core experience index (the WCEI), we may very well have included a few core experiencers among our nonexperiencers category—a state of affairs which, if true, would mean the modest percentages for peacefulness, painlessness, and the absence of fear

TABLE 2

Comparison of Core Experiencers and Nonexperiencers
on the Ten Most Common Affective Reactions
(Ranking Based on Core Experiencers Only)

Characteristic	Core experiencers (n = 49)	Nonexperiencers (n = 53)
Peace	59%	15%
Lack of pain	49%	13%
Lack of fear	47%	9%
Relaxation	29%	4%
Pleasantness	27%	0%
Calmness	20%	6%
Happiness	20%	2%
Joyfulness	20%	0%
Quietude	16%	2%
Warmth	16%	0%

in the later category are somewhat inflated. In fact, most of the statements of peace from the nonexperiencer category (viz., 6 or 8) come from one subgroup—female suicide attempt cases—and appear to reflect more of a sense of relief that their lives were (apparently) over than a feeling of transcendent peace such as was expressed by core experiencers cited earlier. Finally, what is implied in this table is that whereas only one core experiencer failed to report any feelings or emotions, fully thirty-five (or 66 percent) of the nonexperiencers disclosed or implied that they experienced none. Thus, the modal feeling or emotion for the nonexperiencers was—nothing.

Summing up the results of this affective analysis, it is evident that there is a consistent and dramatically positive emotional response to apparent near-death by core experiencers whereas an absence of any affective response is typical for the nonexperiencers. The core experiencers often report overwhelming feelings of peace as well as a transcendent sense of well-being. The nonexperiencers, for the most part, are not conscious of having experienced any emotions during their near-death episodes.

Before concluding this subsection, it may be worthwhile to mention that no person in our sample—including, of course, all our suicide attempt cases—recounted an experience which could be regarded as "a journey to hell." This is consistent with the findings of other large scale studies (e.g., Moody, 1975; Sabom, 1978). Although some near-death experiences did contain frightening aspects or involved moments of confusion and uncertainty, none were characterized by predominantly unpleasant affect or imagery.

Body Separation: Leaving the Body Behind

The second stage of the core experience involves a sense of detachment from one's physical body. As can be seen from Figure 1, about three-eights (37 percent) of our sample reached this stage. Most of these persons report a sense of complete detachment from their bodies though they usually admit they couldn't be sure or weren't actually able to see themselves. In addition, however, sixteen persons in our sample did state that they had distinct and usually clear out-of-the-body experiences. (This figure represents approximately one-third of all those reporting a near-death experience.) Although these accounts vary somewhat, it is typical at this stage in the experience for the individual to find himself/herself in the room looking down on his or her physical body. Most of those reporting this phenomenon commented that somehow they found all this very natural (at the time) and were aware of very acute hearing and sharp but detached mental processes. Visually, the environment is often described as very brightly illuminated.

I shall now recount representative descriptions of various levels of body separation. At the most minimal level, respondents reported either no sense of bodily connection or body awareness. A suicide attempt victim commented:

Mostly it was like a real floating sensation. I don't remember seeing anything. It's real weird. It's like I was detached from everything that was happening. But I didn't see me.

A man who had suffered cardiac arrest related his experience as follows:

It seemed like I was up there in space and just my mind was active. No body feeling, just like my brain was up in space. I had nothing but my mind. Weightless, I had nothing.

The woman who had a cardiac arrest while undergoing a tonsillectomy reported:

I was above. I don't know above what. But I was [pause] up... it was like [pause] like I didn't have a body! I was [pause] but it was me. Not a body, but me! You know what I mean?... It was a me inside. The real me was up there; not this here [pointing to her physical body].

Most commonly, an individual having an out-of-body experience would simply state that he or she was aware of seeing his or her body as though viewing it from outside and above its physical locus—often from an elevated corner of the room or from the ceiling. The following comments are typical accounts of this experience.

The young man who nearly died of a high fever said:

I experienced this type of feeling where I felt I had left my body and I had viewed it from the other side of the room. I can sort of remember looking back at myself—it was scary of course.... I can remember seeing myself lying there with a sheet and a hypothermia blanket on me. My eyes were closed, my face was very cold looking.... It was like I was perched right up on a little level over near the side of the room.... I would be at the foot of the bed, but kind of more up onto the wall, closer to the ceiling, almost in the corner of the room.

A woman who nearly died while giving birth to her second child described her out-of-body experience this way:

I was up in the left-hand corner of the room, looking down at what was going on. ["Could you see clearly?"] I could see very clearly, yeah, yeah. I recognized it as being me. I had absolutely no fear whatsoever. That is one thing that is very definite, that there was no fear.

A woman who had a very serious automobile accident told me that while in a coma:

I had what I term a weird experience. It's where my husband was in the [hospital] room, it was very late at night and I remember looking at the clock—out of my body. It was 11:10 PM and it was where I was looking down at my body; I was actually out of it! ["Did you have any difficulty recognizing yourself?"] Nope. ["How did you look?"] Very pale. Just lying there, arms outstretched, the I.V. in. I can remember a nurse coming in and tucking in the blankets and everything and making sure I was all right and everything. And my hair was all over the pillow. ["Where were 'you' in relation to your physical body?"] I was, like, over in the corner, and being able to watch people walk in the door and being able to see my husband sitting here [she later implies that she felt that she was "up" as well as to one side of her bed].

A man, also badly injured in an automobile crash, remembered a point when:

> At that time I viewed myself from the corner of my hospital room, looking down at my body which was very dark and gray. All the life looked like it was out of it. And my mother was sitting in a chair next to my bed looking very determined and strong in her faith. And my Italian girlfriend at the time was crying at the foot of my bed.

These several accounts of what might be termed, with no pejoration intended, "garden variety" out-of-body experiences will be sufficient, I think, to suggest the subjective locus of the observer relative to his/her body. This sense of elevation was a typical feature in the out-of-body descriptions of my respondents. There were, however, certain other features, thus far unmentioned, which occurred often enough in these accounts to warrant illustration here. One of these features had to do with the quality of illumination present.

The fever victim recalls:

> I can remember it being very, very bright, very bright, and also a very, very peaceful mellow feeling that I had. ["Was the brightness from the illumination in the room?"] No, I don't think so, because, like I said, it was a private room and it had only one window that had a building next to it, so there wasn't much light coming in and I don't think the lighting in the room at that time was that bright. I remember it being very bright. And, like I said, that in combination with a very peaceful, mellow feeling.

During an operation to remove part of his stomach, another man suffered a heart stoppage. He said:

> I remember being up in the air looking down... and seeing myself on the operating table with all the people around working on me. I can remember, what sticks out in my mind mostly, were the colors. Everything in that operating room was a very brilliant, bright color.

Another woman who nearly died in childbirth said:

> As I recall, everything seemed to be brighter. Everything seemed to be lighter and brighter.

The unusual brightness of the environment was, thus, one

noteworthy aspect of the out-of-body experience for several respondents. Another such feature, commented on by at least three respondents, was the sense of viewing oneself as though from a great height.

> I seemed to be very high in the air. The people I was looking at were rather small. I couldn't tell you how high I was, but I was up, and I seemed to be looking through a hole in a cloud. It was like rainbows, it was bright rays shining down.
>
> It seemed like my body was further away. I seemed to be higher than the ceiling.

Another woman who nearly lost her life in an automobile accident recalled her out-of-body perception as follows:

> Even though I was very close physically to the doctors, they seemed to be very far away while I was watching them operate on me.

A final feature of these out-of-body experiences which requires comment has to do with what may be called the "mind-state" which accompanies them. The protocols I have already cited have mentioned several emotional reactions ranging from initial fear to the total absence of fear; we have also had indications here of a delicious sense of peacefulness. Nevertheless, from a reading of all the relevant protocols, the feature which clearly stands out as typical of the mind-state of out-of-body experiencers is the sense of observer-like detachment, often associated with a feeling that "all this is perfectly natural." Some illustrative quotes follow.

> Mostly, I think I was just observing.... It didn't feel as though it was happening to me at all. I was just the observer.

A young woman who nearly died of complications resulting from a faulty exploratory surgery procedure stated:

> I was totally objective. I was just an onlooker. I was just viewing things and just taking it in. But I was making no judgments—just waiting, I guess. Just waiting to die and just realizing that all these things were going on.... I was the classic "fly on the wall." I was just there.
>
> It was as if I was supposed to be watching it. It was part of what you were supposed to do...it seemed very natural.
>
> It seemed perfectly right. Everything about it seemed right. Perfectly natural.

It seemed very [pause] it seemed like it was the thing to do....It wasn't a problem to me.

In order to avoid a possible point of confusion, it is necessary to emphasize that all of the persons whose remarks I've just cited also reported the core experience affective response of peace and a sense of well-being. The affective response itself usually pervades the entire experience. The psychological mind-state of detached observation or reflection is typical chiefly of the out-of-body stage of the experience.

The genuineness of apparent out-of-body perceptions is, of course, an important issue, but space limitations preclude our considering it here. Suffice it to say that there was, in at least a couple of my cases, suggestive evidence of such genuineness. Such examples, in any event, have already been furnished by other near-death researchers (e.g., Moody, 1975; Sabom and Kreutziger, 1978; Rawlings, 1978).

Entering the Darkness

The next stage of the experience seems to be a transitional one between this world and whatever may be said to lie beyond. I call it "entering the darkness." This space is usually characterized as completely black or dark, very peaceful, and, at least in the majority of such accounts, without dimension. Most persons have the sense of floating or drifting through it, though a few respondents reported that they felt they were moving very rapidly through this space.

Figure 1 demonstrates that slightly less than one-quarter (23 percent) of our sample encounter this feature of the core experience.

Moody's (1975) work implied that many individuals experience this phenomenon as travelling through a dark tunnel. We found some evidence for this interpretation, but only among a minority of our respondents who "entered the darkness." Specifically, nine persons described their experience in ways consistent with the Moody tunnel paradigm. These respondents did in fact choose the word "tunnel" most frequently to designate the space they found themselves in, although occasionally other similar terms were used (e.g., funnel, pipe, culvert, and drum).

A woman who suffered a cerebral hemorrhage and temporary blindness told me:

I remember going through a tunnel, a very, very dark tunnel....["Did you feel the tunnel was vast?"] Yes, very, very. It started at a narrow point and became wider and wider. But I remember it being very, very black. But even though it was black, I wasn't afraid because I knew that there was something at the other end waiting for me that was good.... I found it very pleasant. I wasn't afraid or anything. There was no fear attached to it. I felt very light. I felt like I was floating.

Another woman who almost died during open heart surgery remembered:

I was—it was a great big drum and this drum was black. In my mind I says, "The Bible says we walk through a dark tunnel until we reach light." And I says, "When am I going to reach the light?" ["You felt you were in the tunnel?"] I was in the tunnel, yeah. I was in this great big tunnel and I walked and I walked and I walked and I says, "When am I going to see the light? I'm dead, but when am I going to see the light?" ["You felt you were dead?"] I was dead, yeah.... It seemed like [pause] there was no light. I never saw the light.

A young woman who experienced a near fatal asthma attack observed:

I do remember thinking to myself that I was dying. And I felt I was floating through a tunnel.... When I say "tunnel," the only thing I can think of is—you know those sewer pipes, those big pipes they put in? It was round like that, but it was enormous. I couldn't really see the edges of it; I got the feeling that it was round. It was like a whitish color. I was just smack in the middle. My whole body, you know. I was lying on my back. I was just floating. And smoke or white lines or something were coming this way [toward her] and I was going the opposite way. ["What kind of feeling did you have as you were floating through this tunnel?"] Very peaceful, almost as if I were on a raft in the ocean, you know?

More commonly, the experience of "entering the darkness" was phrased in terms of a journey into a black vastness without shape or dimension. An account which is seemingly a combination of the tunnel and the black dimensionless domain comes from a woman who experienced an immediate post-delivery embolism.

It's just like a void, a nothing and it's such a peaceful—it's so pleasant that you can keep going. It's a complete blackness, there is no sensation at all, there was no feeling. ["Did it have any kind of form to it?"] No—sort of like a dark tunnel. Just a floating. It's like [being] in mid-air.

More typical expressions of this dark dimensionless space are given next.

A young man, badly injured in a motorcycle crash, relates:

> I felt as though I was—well, that's the hard part to explain—like you're floating. Like you're there and, believe it or not, the color is—there is no color [pause], it's like a darkness. ["Did the darkness have a shape of any kind?"] It was empty. Yeah, that's it. Space. Just nothing. Nothing but something. It's like trying to describe the end of the universe.

An eighteen-year-old man, intent on committing suicide by jumping from a cliff in midwinter, lost his footing and sustained a head injury resulting in unconsciousness. While unconscious he found himself in

> ...a darkness, it was a very darkness...it was a total nothing.

The woman who suffered cardiac arrest during a tonsillectomy recalled:

> Well, it was like night. It was dark. It was dark. But it was like, like [pause] like in the dark sky. Space. Dark. And it was—there weren't any things around. No stars or objects around.

The woman whose remarks I cited earlier to illustrate the affective tone of the core experience may be quoted again in the present content:

> I think that the next thing I remember is total, peaceful, wonderful blackness. Very peaceful blackness. [She then heard her name called as though from a great distance.] I remember distinctly thinking to myself how easy it would be to slip back into that nice peaceful blackness. [Afterward, while still in the hospital, she was intensely happy, so much so that people commented on it.] My happiness had no connection with the fact that I was alive again; my happiness seemed at that time to be connected with that total peaceful blackness.

Finally, let me quote a woman whose case is most unusual in our sample for two reasons. First, she had recurrent near-death episodes—she estimates twelve to fourteen of them—as a child between the ages of nine and sixteen, as a result of heart stoppages resulting from rheumatic fever. Second, since at the time of her interview, she was a woman in her mid-fifties, she was describing experiences that, in some cases, took place nearly half a century before! Needless to say, reasonable questions can be raised concerning the accuracy of her recall of these childhood memories. She herself emphatically averred that the form of her experience was identical on the occasion of each such near-fatal episode. However that may be, her observations here are of some interest if only because they seem to square with other, much more recent, accounts:

> [During these attacks she would reach a point where she would] go over is the only—descend into this feeling of soft velvet blackness. It wasn't like going into a tunnel [she had recently read Moody's first book]; I had no feeling of going into a tunnel. I just seemed to be surrounded by a velvet blackness and a softness and I would have absolutely no fear and the pain would disappear when I entered into this other state.

Whether the experience is recognized as floating through a dark tunnel or entering a black spaceless void, it is clear that those individuals who have reached this stage of the core experience have begun to encounter very nonordinary realms of consciousness. In fact, what I have so far related is scarcely more than a prelude to a set of phenomena which are themselves so extraordinary in character that they require an interruption of this sequential narrative of the core experience in order to do them justice.

Certain events appear to be decisive in determining whether an individual is to return from the journey on which his near-death episode has launched him.

At the Crossroads: The Decisional Process

For the majority of the core experiencers, there is a point in their passage toward (apparent) death when they become aware that a decision has to be made concerning their future: Are they to return to life or continue on toward death? Awareness of reaching this decisional choice point is usually signalled by one of several remarkable phenomenological features. I shall list them here and then provide detailed case histories to illustrate them. Because of their similarity from case to case, these features, taken in their totality, are unquestionably among the most provocative of the elements regularly associated with the core experience.

1. The life review. The individual may experience all of his life or selected aspects of it in the form of very vivid and nearly instantane-

ous visual images. These images usually appear in no definite sequence (though they sometimes do), but rather as a simultaneous matrix of impressions, like a hologram. In some instances, they appear to include flashforwards as well as flashbacks. They are usually overwhelmingly positive in affective tone, even though the individual viewing them ordinarily (but not always) experiences them with a sense of detachment. Twelve persons—or about one-fourth of our core experiencer sample—reported this phenomenon.

2. The encounter with "a presence." Sometimes in association with the life review feature, sometimes independently of it, the individual may become aware of what I shall call here "a presence."[5] My respondents never reported actually seeing the presence; rather, they always sensed or inferred it. On occasion, however, it was *heard* to speak (though sometimes this was described as a "mental understanding") and then it spoke with a voice that is clearly audible (to the experiencer) and identifiable as to gender.[6] The respondent usually feels as though there is mutual direct communication between the presence and himself/herself. Although there is some variation, the presence usually states or implies that the individual is at a choice-point in his life and that it is up to him/her to decide whether to return (i.e., to physical life). At this point the individual seems led either to reflect on his/her life or to re-experience it in the form of the panoramic life review imagery just described, as he/she attempts to make up his/her mind. In some cases, the individual seems to be given information about his/her future physical existence, if he/she should decide to live. Altogether, twenty persons in our sample—or slightly more than two-fifths of our core experiencers—indicated that they were aware of what I have called a presence.[7]

3. The encounter with deceased loved ones. In a few cases—there were eight clear instances of this—the respondent becomes aware of the "spirits" of deceased loved ones, usually relatives. In contrast to the phenomenon of the "presence," these "spirits" are usually seen and recognized.[8] Typically, they greet the individual in a friendly fashion while the respondent himself/herself usually experiences a combination of surprise and great happiness at this apparent reunion. Nevertheless, these spirits usually inform the respondent that, in effect, "it isn't your time" and that "you must go back." Thus, while the "presence" usually appears to give the respondent a choice whether "to stay," the "spirits" usually urge the individual "to

return." This difference between the encounter with a presence and an encounter with spirits, especially when one bears in mind the (near) mutually exclusive relationship between them, suggests that they represent two quite distinct and independent phases of the core experience decisional process.

4. Making the decision. The result of the events just described is a decision made either by or for the individual to return to life or continue further on the journey beyond life. Not surprisingly, virtually all core experiencers feel that either they themselves decided to "come back" or that they were "sent back" (in a few instances, apparently, against their own preferences). Sixteen persons—about one-third of our core experiencers—testified that they either chose, bargained, or willed themselves to return. Five persons stated that they felt they were sent back. For the remaining respondents—seven in number—who appear to have experienced at least one aspect of the decisional process how the decision was made is not clear. In a few cases, however, a decision was apparently arrived at by an individual without any of the three features described above occurring in a clear-cut fashion.

Whether the individual feels he or she chose to return or was sent back, the reasons given usually have to do with one or the other of two nonindependent considerations: (1) the "pull" of loved ones—usually children or spouses—who are felt to have need of the respondent or (2) a sense that one's life's tasks and purposes are not yet accomplished—a feeling of "unfinished business."

In any case, the reaching of a decision is usually the last event of which a core experiencer has any recollection. The decision appears to reverse the dying process and returns the individual to the world of ordinary reality.

The components comprising the decison process manifest themselves during various stages of the core experience. They may in fact appear in connection with any of the stages of the core experience (since they crosscut these stages), but they tend to occur in association with either the out-of-body or the entering-the-darkness stages, or with the stage to be described in the next section. Altogether, by a conservative count, twenty-eight core experiencers (or 57 percent) appear to have passed through a decisional phase; nineteen in a very marked and obvious way; and the remainder to various lesser degrees.

In order to recreate the sense of these complex decisional

episodes, it will be necessary here to reproduce some lengthy extracts from our interviews, as much as possible in their full context.

The following conversation was with a respondent who was involved in a motorcycle accident at the age of eighteen.

RESPONDENT: During the time I was supposedly dead—according to them [the doctors], supposedly I was dead—during this time it was like I was talking to someone that—I never knew who they were; that was strange. I asked, but I never got an answer. The only thing I can remember is like a voice says, "Well, you've made it. You've finally made it." I says, "No, this is too early. What are you talking about?" He says, "Well, you've finally left; you don't have to suffer anymore." I had been sick as a kid and it hurt. And he says, "You don't have to suffer anymore. You made it." I says, "What do you mean? I want to go back. I can't [pause] I can't—I haven't done anything. I'm still trying to go to school. And work. I've got people that need me. And things I've *got* to do. A lot of unfinished things that I've got to do. And I'd like to go back—if that's possible." And then the voice says, "Well, it's up to you. If you go back, you're going to suffer because you're really hurt. You're going to suffer. And you're going to have to endure some real pain." [Indeed, the respondent reports having suffered intense pain for the next year during his recuperation.] And I says, "Well, it doesn't matter to me. That I can handle. Just let me go back." And they said, "Well, okay." And at that instant, I felt a drop of water hit my—and then the doctor screamed, "He's alive, he's alive!"

INTERVIEWER: Do you remember being aware of any unusual noises or sounds?

RESPONDENT: The only sound I was aware of was the voice. And it sounded—it seemed to be a man's voice. It seemed to be soft, yet harsh.

INTERVIEWER: Were you aware of any other persons, voices, presences?

RESPONDENT: Just one. Just the one voice and it was like an entrance.

INTERVIEWER: Like an entrance?

RESPONDENT: Yeah, it was like a walk-in person. Like a voice that says—like a greeting voice. Or like, "Well, here you are. You finally made it."

INTERVIEWER: Now this wasn't a voice of anyone that you recognize—anyone in your family?

RESPONDENT: No. This is why I tried to describe it as being a harsh voice yet soft—but sure.

INTERVIEWER: You said before [referring to a portion of the interview not quoted here] that you kind of felt reassured when you heard this voice.

RESPONDENT: Comforting. It was a comforting voice.

INTERVIEWER: It essentially said, "You've made it now. You're not going to have any more pain." And then you kind of bargained to get back.

RESPONDENT: Right. It gave me a choice. I had a choice of staying or going back.

The next dialogue is with the woman who suffered cardiac arrest during a tonsillectomy. According to her own account, she was told afterward that she was "clinically dead" for nearly three minutes.[9] At this point in the interview, the respondent is describing her sense of "being up," i.e., elevated in space.

RESPONDENT: And I was *above*. And there was—a presence. It's the only way I can explain it—because I didn't see anything. But there was [pause] a presence and it may not have been talking to me, but it was, it was like [pause] like I knew what was going on between our minds.

INTERVIEWER: Sort of like telepathy?

RESPONDENT: Well, I guess so. It wasn't that I remember him telling me that I had to go down, but it was as if I knew I had to go down. And I didn't want to. Yet I wanted to. And it was like being pulled without being pulled. My feelings I guess were [pause] pulled apart. I wasn't afraid to go that way. This is the only way I can explain it. I wasn't afraid to go that way. I wanted to go that way. I really did.

INTERVIEWER: In this upward direction?

RESPONDENT: That way there [pointing upward, on a diagonal]. I wanted to go there. Something was there. I remember that there was something there—a presence there. And I had no fear of it. And the peace, the *release* [pause], the fear was all gone. There was no pain. There was nothing. It was just absolutely beautiful! I could never explain it in a million years. It was a feeling that I think everybody dreams of someday having. Reaching a point of *absolute* peace. To me peace is the greatest word that I can express. That's all I can really remember—that I was being drawn back. It was a choice, evidently that I made.

INTERVIEWER: Do you feel that you made the choice?

RESPONDENT: Yes, I think so. I wasn't afraid to go that way. And yet I'm sure it was my choice to come back.

INTERVIEWER: Why do you feel you came back? Why did you choose to come back?

RESPONDENT: I don't know. I think it's because I had two little children. And I felt they needed me more than—up there. And I think going up there meant my peace and joy, but it meant misery for my children. And I think even then I was thinking of these things—weighing things. I wasn't feeling any pain or sorrow or anything, but I was thinking calmly and rationally, making a decision—a rational decision, a logical decision— without emotions involved. Do you know what I mean? I didn't make that decision emotionally. I made it logically. And the choice, both choices were—I mean, I wasn't afraid to die so that choice would have been just as easy for me. But the choice was made logically. And I'm sure it was mine.

In the following instance, the respondent is unusual in that he reports that his experience came back to him bit by bit, like fragments of a forgotten dream, only after several years had passed since his near-death episode, brought about by an automobile accident.

RESPONDENT: It was like I got to view my whole life as a movie, and see it and get to view different things that happened, different things that took place. [pause] I think I got to see some things in the future; I might even have gotten to see how my whole life might have turned out or will turn out—I don't know—as far as the future destiny of it. It's hard to say. Sometimes I recognize things when I get there and go, Wow! So anyway, I got to see, basically, what was a whole view of my life. Now, after I was shown a lot of things which somehow it's very hard on words on describing...basically, it was like watching a movie. But this movie, although it is speeded up, probably to show you it all—it only seems to take a second—and the next thing was a voice coming to me after all this and saying, very compassionately, it was like an all-knowing voice, something that at the time I took to be the voice of Jesus, but I can take it to be the voice of any one God as far as the whole universe is concerned. I don't know who that person was. It was like a voice that I knew and it said to me, "You really blew it this time, Frank."

INTERVIEWER: Did it actually use those words?

RESPONDENT: Yes. Actual words, "You really blew it this time, Frank." Right there it was like I was shown this movie and then the voice said that to me—and at that time I viewed myself from the corner of my hospital room, looking down at my body which was very dark and gray. All the life looked like it was out of it. And my mother was sitting in a chair next to my bed looking very determined and strong in her faith. And my Italian girlfriend at the time was crying at the foot of my bed—in beautiful form—it was beautiful. But, anyway, at this time the voice said, "You really blew it this time, Frank." And I looked down at this scene and that scene compared with the fact that I had seen this view of my life and I said, "No! I want to live." And at that saying, it was almost like, it seems like, it was a snap [he snaps his fingers] and I was sort of inside my body. And the next thing—was waking up and looking down at my girlfriend and saying, "Jesus Christ, it's bad enough that I'm dying and you got to sit there and cry!" [He laughs.]

I shall cite one more case along these lines primarily to illustrate the nature of the communication between the presence/voice and the individual. This material is drawn from the interview with the young man who accidentally knocked himself unconscious as he was on the threshold of suicide.

RESPONDENT: The first thing was, when I was out, I had a really weird feeling like [pause] I was going somewhere. I don't know where I was going but [trails off]...I don't know where I was going but I was moving to an emptiness. And then, all of a sudden, I heard this voice. And it was a really, a really [pause] calm; and it was just a great—it was a male voice. It was just really great. It was just a really—like someone talking to me as a real close friend or something like that. It was a really nice tone of voice, you know what I mean?

INTERVIEWER: Compassionate?

RESPONDENT: Yeah. It was great. Yeah. And, and, the first thing he said was, "Do you really want to die?" And I said, "Yes. Nothing has been going right all my life and at this point I really don't care if I live or die." And he says, "What about your mother? She cares about you. What about your girlfriend?" And then it got kind of hazy and he said something about a daughter but—I don't have a daughter! So I think it's sort of like, like, you know, sometime in the near future I'm going to have a daughter and she's going to be something important, because if God wants me to live, there must be some purpose in my life. And my daughter is going to be something important— maybe she'll find a cure for cancer or maybe she'll [pause]— something like that. Or make something very important like— maybe she'll solve ecological problems or maybe the population or something very important that will help prolong the existence of mankind which is coming very short, you know? And so, anyhow, then he said, "Do you want to go back?" and I says, "What do you mean, go back?" And he goes, "Finish your life on earth." And I go, "No. I want to die." And he goes, "You are breaking my laws to commit suicide. You'll not be with me in Heaven—if you die." And I says, "What will happen?" And then after this I started coming to. So I don't know what happened after this. So I think that God was trying to tell me that if I commit suicide I'm going to Hell, you know? So, I'm not going to think about suicide any more. [Nervous laughter.]

Further into the interview, the respondent offered some illuminating observations concerning how the voice of the presence is experienced. His comments here are, to the best of my knowledge, very indicative of the form that this kind of "communication" takes in most cases.

INTERVIEWER: Okay, let's focus on the voice then. You never saw anything?

RESPONDENT: No, it was still. The whole time it was in complete darkness.

INTERVIEWER: Even during the time that the voice was speaking to you?

RESPONDENT: Yeah.

INTERVIEWER: When you heard the voice, you heard it as a male voice. Did you actually hear the words, or—

RESPONDENT: It was like it was coming into my mind. It was like I didn't have any hearing or any sight or anything. It was like it was projected into my mind.

INTERVIEWER: What you told me before—is that the gist of what the voice said? Or is it pretty much the actual words?

RESPONDENT: It was mostly thoughts, you know? It was mostly thoughts. It wasn't like somebody—you know, like you and I are communicating with words. It was mostly thoughts—like, I would picture in my mind my mother crying and my girlfriend crying and then when there was the thought about a daughter, she [his girlfriend] was holding a baby. It was like—the more I think over it, the more it comes out as words, but when it happened it was more like symbols—symbolic, you know?

INTERVIEWER: So what you're doing now is trying to translate it into words?

RESPONDENT: I'm trying to change it into English, yeah. It was very specific.

INTERVIEWER: But the message to you was very clear?

RESPONDENT: Yes. It was very clear. That my life isn't ended yet and that I shouldn't be trying to fool around with my life because it isn't under my control, you know?

In some cases, as I have mentioned, an individual is enjoined to return to life by the exhortations of a "visible spirit" rather than an "audible presence." To conclude this section, I shall give just one example of this mode of resolution of an individual's near-death crisis.

In this case, a woman, while hospitalized, was experiencing severe respiratory problems due to a chronic asthmatic condition. She had been feeling extremely uncomfortable, unable to breathe, move or talk, but then became aware that she was feeling comfortable. Apparently without moving, she saw a room monitor go flat.

I thought, "Gee, I feel so comfortable." And then I heard, I heard Mrs. Friedrich [a wealthy woman for whom the respondent had once worked; the respondent described Mrs. Friedrich as a very loving and much respected woman; she, herself, loved her and felt loved by her]. She had been dead for nine years at that time. I heard, in her very distinct voice—she spoke slowly and every word was brought out strong—and she had a low voice, and she said, "Miss Harper... *Miss Harper*... MISS HARPER [with gradually increasing volume and emphasis], I want you to live." And she appeared, not distinctly, but... it's hard to explain... I don't think I saw her face; it was there but it was more of a [leaves off] she was dressed in black. I don't think I could see her feet, but I could see the middle part of her, and it was almost as if you would look at the side of a tree, a straight tree. And I saw this simple black dress and it just sort of faded out, top and bottom. But she was there and she said, "Miss Harper. Miss Harper! I want you to live!"[This was repeated many times.] And she said, "I didn't build this hospital for my family to die in; I built this hospital so that my family could live!" She said it many times and distinctly. It was the wing of the hospital she had built. And finally I answered in my mind, "I'll try, Mrs. Friedrich, I'll try"[said weakly]. And she said [forcibly] "Miss Harper. Miss Harper! I want you to live!"

It is tempting to quote from additional interviews to illustrate further nuances of the decisional process, but perhaps enough case history material has already been cited to convey something of the sense of awe, wonder, comfort, and peace that usually accompanies the decision to return to life. It will be obvious from the excerpts presented in this section that the decision to return to life is usually made in an atmosphere that has a very definite other-worldly ambiance. A specifically religious interpretation is given to it by many, though not all, of the core experiencers. However this might be, the interpretive questions must be eschewed here in order to return to our narrative account of the stages of the near-death experience. For individuals who fail to undergo any conscious decisional crisis by stage 3 there may be further aspects of the experience of dying which present themselves next—and these we must now consider.

Seeing the Light

The passage from the third to the fourth stage of the core experience is marked by one singular feature: the appearance of light. It is usually described as a brilliant golden light. This light, however, almost never hurts one's eyes but is, on the contrary, very restful and comforting and, apparently, of ineffable beauty.[10] Some of my respondents told me that they felt enveloped by this light and virtually all who experienced it felt drawn to it. Occasionally the light is associated with the phenomenon of the sensed presence, discussed in the last subsection, but this is by no means always the case. Figure 1 shows that sixteen persons—or about one-third of our core experiencers—reported seeing this kind of light.

For many respondents, though not all, the golden light brings to an end the "time of darkness" and thus seems to signal an entirely new stage of the experience. In the midst of at least some of my respondents, the transition from darkness to light is packed with symbolic meaning: phenomenologically, if not ontologically, it is taken to signify the termination of the experience of dying and the beginning of new life. Of course, for religiously-minded individuals the golden light is sometimes taken to be the visual manifestation of God and two of my respondents appear to have had a vision of Jesus in connection with their near-death incident, in which he was surrounded by this light.

As usual, to illustrate the phenomena typical of this stage, we turn directly to our interview protocols.

Sometimes the transition from darkness to light is stated very simply, as it was by the woman who had recurrent near-death episodes as a child:

I just seemed to be surrounded by a velvet blackness, and then, sort of at the periphery of the velvet blackness, there was a brilliant golden light. And I don't remember feeling frightened at all, just perfectly at peace and perfectly comfortable as if this is where I should be.

In some cases, the transition from darkness to light is associated with the presence as it was in the following example when a voice told the respondent that she was being sent back:

It was dark and it was like—hard to believe—like you were going from dark to light. I can't explain it...all of a sudden there was light. And then when the voice was coming to me...it was just like light. [Was the light bright?] Not piercingly. [Did it hurt your eyes?] No.

In other cases, the light is described in a more detailed way and in a definite "tunnel context." The following material is taken from an account of a seventy-year-old woman who was in ill health at the time I interviewed her. She had had a near-death episode stemming from a respiratory failure two years earlier. After having had an out-of-body experience, she said, mentally, to herself:

I'm going to go over to the other side. There's a culvert over there. I want to go through [to] see what's in that culvert. I can see the culvert

now. It was just like one of these big water culverts. Great big one.
But when I went over there and walked into it, I could stand up. And
I says, geez, that's funny, I never could when I was a kid. We'd crawl
through them. Here I could stand up and walk. And as I started to
walk, I saw this beautiful, golden light, way, way small, down the
tunnel. I said that's a funny light. It doesn't even look like gold and
yet it is gold and it isn't yellow. I'll go see what's on the other side.
Maybe it—it must be pretty over there. And I kept thinking, well,
yeah, I'll go, I'll go see.

Another illustration of the magnetic pull of the light is taken from
the testimony of a woman who had a cardiac arrest. She found
herself walking down a path:

and as I was walking down...there was a wee bit of a light down at
the extreme end of it and as I kept walking down, that light kept
getting brighter and brighter all the time. Really, it was beautiful
while it lasted, but it was such a short time, because then they gave me
a shot...and I was out.

In other instances, as I have already indicated, the light does not
merely beckon from a distance, but appears to enfold the individual
in what can only be described as a "loving way." The following
examples will serve to justify this subjective-sounding characterization.

INTERVIEWER: Were you ever aware at any point of a light or glow
or any kind of illumination?
RESPONDENT: A light glow. There was a glow.
INTERVIEWER: Was it in the room itself, or was it somewhere else?
RESPONDENT: In the room.
INTERVIEWER: Different from the illumination that was provided
naturally?
RESPONDENT: Oh, yes. Different, very different. It was like
[pause] a tawny gold. It was just like on the outer ridges of
where I was at. It was just like me looking through—and being
apart from everything and just looking. And it was really,
really [pause] I felt warm from that.
INTERVIEWER: So that was a positive aspect?
RESPONDENT: It was peaceful. I can remember it being very, very
bright, very bright, and also a very, very peaceful, mellow
feeling that I had.

INTERVIEWER: Was the brightness from the illumination in the room?

RESPONDENT: No, I don't think so, because, as I said, it was a private room and it had only one window that had a building next to it, so there wasn't much light coming in and I don't think the lighting in the room at that time was that bright. I remember it being very bright. And, like I said, that in combination with a very peaceful, mellow feeling.

INTERVIEWER: Tell me more about the light.

RESPONDENT: Very, very bright, like the sun was right in my room shining down. And it seemed like, if there was any color, all the colors were their brightest. You know, everything just magnified a lot of light, it seems like.

INTERVIEWER: Did the brightness of the colors hurt your eyes?

RESPONDENT: No, I could just see the colors so perfectly.

INTERVIEWER: What did you make of this?

RESPONDENT: Well, I look at the whole thing as being like a kind of utopia. Like this is the way the colors are in utopia, perfect. Perfect to their natural color.

RESPONDENT: I had the sensation of warm, a very warm sensation, of a very [pause] it was like a light. You know, I can't explain it, what the light looks like, but it has a very—and I can see it, just like I'm going through it right now—like a very warm, comforting light that I had. And it wasn't centered on anything; it was, like, all around me. It was all around me.

INTERVIEWER: It enveloped you?

RESPONDENT: Right! It was all around me. And the colors, the colors, were very vivid—very vivid colors. I had a feeling of total peace. A feeling of total, total peace. Tremendous peace. Tremendous peace. In fact, I just lay there—my bed was right near the window—and I remembered I stared out the window— and the light, and everything, was even outside!

INTERVIEWER: Did that light hurt your eyes?

RESPONDENT: No.

INTERVIEWER: Was it bright?

RESPONDENT: No. Not bright, it was not bright. It was like a shaded lamp or something. But it wasn't that kind of light that you get from a lamp. You know what it was? Like someone had put a shade over the sun. It had me feel very, very peaceful. I was no longer afraid. Everything was going to be all right.

The various manifestations of the light which I have reviewed here brings us to the threshold of the last stage of the core experience, as suggested by my data. From this point on, the light serves no longer primarily either as a beacon or as a warm, enveloping effulgence. Instead, it becomes the preternatural illumination of what my respondents perceive as the world beyond death.

Entering the Light

The difference between the preceding stage and this one is the difference between seeing the light and entering into "a world" in which the light appears to have its origin. For, according to the reports indicative of having reached this stage, one does indeed have the sense of being in another world—and it is a world of preternatural beauty. The colors are said to be unforgettable. The individual may find himself/herself in a meadow or see unusual physical-like structures which, however, do not seem to correspond exactly to anything in our world. This is the stage where felt presences are seen. It is, in fact, typically "here" where respondents report being greeted by deceased relatives. Five persons claimed to have seen beautiful flowers here and four were aware of hearing lovely music. Although resentment at being brought back from imminent death was not frequently expressed by our respondents, that sentiment was particularly evident in several persons who were "returned to life" after experiencing this stage.

Figure 1 reveals that only ten persons—or about one-fifth of our core experience sample—gave evidence of penetrating this final stage. Indeed, it is typically the case—at least among my respondents—that only a glimpse, rather than a protracted visit, is vouchsafed those who come this far. One person whose experience and reaction were representative of this group said that she was afforded "just a peek" into what she felt was "the hereafter." Accordingly, with only a few exceptions, the descriptions we have of this domain tend to be decidedly and perhaps disappointingly sketchy.

Unfortunately, though the few more extensive descriptions of this stage are among the most provocative of my case history materials, space limitations preclude my presenting them. Instead, to summarize this stage, I shall have to draw on a few brief accounts.

From a cardiac arrest victim:

I happened to go down this path and it was beautiful. Beautiful flowers and the birds were singing, and I was walking down. [After she was resuscitated] I did reprimand my surgeon and my cardiologist. I said, "Why, in heaven's name did you bring me back? It was so beautiful."

From a woman who suffered a respiratory failure:

I was in a field, a large empty field, and it had high, golden grass that was very soft, so bright. And my pain was gone and it was quiet, but it wasn't a morbid quiet, it was a peaceful quiet. [Afterward] I said to Dr. _____, "why did you bring me back?" I didn't want to come back. So I was really very happy in that place, wherever it was. [She later further described the field she found herself in.] Soft, silky, very brilliant gold. [The light was] just bright, but restful. The grass swayed. It was very peaceful, very quiet. The grass was so outstandingly beautiful that I will never forget it.

A man who appears to have come close to dying as a result of being ill during a tooth extraction[11] gave the following statement:

I took a trip to heaven. I saw the most beautiful lakes. Angels—they were floating around like you see seagulls. Everything was white. The most beautiful flowers. Nobody on this earth ever saw the beautiful flowers that I saw there.... I don't believe there is a color on this earth that wasn't included in that color situation that I saw. Everything, everything. Of course, I was so impressed with the beauty of everything there that I couldn't pinpoint any one thing.... Everything was bright. The lakes were blue, light blue. Everything about the angels was pure white. ["Tell me what the angels looked like."] I can't. ["Did the colors hurt your eyes?"] No. ["Was it restful?"] It was. Everything about the whole thing was restful.

A woman who nearly died as a result of a cerebral hemmorrhage described a part of her experience as follows:

There was music, very, very pleasant music:...The music was beautiful....[Later] And then there was another part to it where two aunts of mine—they're dead... and they were sitting on a rail and it was a beautiful meadow and they started calling me. They said, "Come on, Giselle, come on."... And I was very happy to see them— it was a meadow lane, beautiful grass, and they were sitting on this railing and calling me... and I went halfway and then stopped. And that's probably when I came to.

Finally, a woman in her mid-thirties who suffered congestive heart failure during surgery for a chronic intestinal disorder, reported a very deep core experience. She clearly observed her physical body "below" her on the operating table and then suddenly found herself in what she described as a "very pretty valley" during which time she was aware of "awesome, spiritual" music. At this time, she encountered her deceased grandfather who instructed her to return to life, saying that she was "still needed." At this point, I shall quote further from her interview protocol in order to amplify her description and interpretation of her surroundings:

> INTERVIEWER: Could you describe for me a little bit more the valley? You said it was like the valley of the shadow of death.[12] Are there more things that come to mind in terms of what you can recall about it? How you felt? What you were aware of? What you saw?
> RESPONDENT: I think I should say that this Psalm happens to be my favorite Psalm. And while I've never seen the valley of the shadow of death before, it was just a very beautiful, crystal-like place, and it just gave me a very good feeling once I realized where I was.
> INTERVIEWER: And you did have this realization at the time? It wasn't something that you had come to after the experience, but at the time it occurred you said, "this is where I am." Was it like—was it comparable to any place that you've been to? Was it earthly? Was it—
> RESPONDENT: No. It wasn't earthly. I can't say if it was heavenly because I really don't know what heaven is like, but it didn't seem earthly at all.
> INTERVIEWER: Can you say anything about the illumination of the valley? Could you see it clearly?
> RESPONDENT: It was very bright. Very bright.
> INTERVIEWER: Did the bright light hurt your eyes?
> RESPONDENT: No. Not at all.

A casual perusal of all of the accounts presented in this subsection—even those which are very brief—will be sufficient to disclose that each of them, without exception, uses the adjective "beautiful" to describe the sensed features of the "surroundings" where these respondents found themselves. If I may take the liberty of speaking about this realm as a "world" of its own, then, plainly and without equivocation, it is experienced as a beautiful world sans pareil. Reading these accounts, it is understandable why a person entering into such a world would be reluctant, even unwilling, to return to the world of ordinary experience.

Nevertheless, all those persons in my sample who reached the threshold of this world were obliged to return and no one reported venturing into any further realms that might be construed as transcending this one. With the description of this stage of the core experience, then, we have followed the phenomenological path of dying persons as far as these accounts will take us. As Moody has implied, it seems to be the same journey with different individuals encountering different segments of what appears to be a single, common path.

CONCLUSION

Although I have had to limit my presentation largely to a statistical and descriptive rendering of the core experience, I think it will be obvious to the attentive reader that the data I have offered here strongly corroborate those stemming from Moody's informal study. There may be some differences in conceptualization, but there is no mistaking the common underlying pattern of the core experience itself. As other researchers (e.g., Sabom and Kreutziger, 1978; Sabom, 1981; Osis and Haraldsson, 1977; Greyson and Stevenson, 1980) have already begun to furnish still additional independent corroboration for Moody's findings, I think we can now regard the core experience as a well-documented, authentic phenomenon. Our task now would seem to be to address ourselves to such questions as these: (1) What are the conditions which affect the likelihood and depth of the experience? (2) What are the personal and psychological correlates of the core experience? (3) To what extent is the core experience a universal, culture-free phenomenon? (4) How is this phenomenon to be interpreted?

The articles in this volume provide some preliminary answers to these questions, of course, but at this stage in our knowledge our situation is perhaps rather like Galileo's just after he viewed the heavens through his crude telescope. As for him, a new dimension of human existence seems to be opening up to use through scientific inquiry, but we still have much to learn before we can come to see with any clarity just what it is that has apparently been revealed to us and what, ultimately, it may signify.

Notes

1. The author gratefully acknowledges the support provided for this investigation by the University of Connecticut Research Foundation.

2. From this point on, I shall use the term "core (near-death) experience" (Ring, 1980) to designate the prototypic experience described by Moody.

3. Further details of the research procedures and findings of this study are available in my book, *Life at Death.*

4. Sabom and I both used the WCEI and the same cutoff points in analyzing our respective data.

5. This term was used by a number of my respondents and seems as phenomenologically appropriate as any.

6. I did not systematically ask about the gender associated with a presence who spoke until after a couple of respondents volunteered that "it was a man's voice." Altogether, six respondents identified the voice they heard as "a man's voice" or "a male voice." Both from other data in my own sample and informal conversations with near-death survivors not part of this study, however, I would not want to claim that the voice is *always* heard as masculine. Obviously, the number of cases involved here is far too small for any generalizations to be based on them. This is a question for further research.

7. In a few cases here counted as positive, the respondent did not actually use the term "presence" or "person" or "God" to represent the external source of the communication, but the phenomenological features associated with this event were otherwise in keeping with the description given here.

8. In fact, the experience of the presence and that of encountering deceased loved ones were almost always mutually exclusive—a respondent would encounter either one or the other, *but not both.* The sole exception to this pattern is that of a woman who felt that she "had a conversation with God" but who also claimed to have had a vague sense of deceased others. Her perception of the latter, however, was very indistinct compared to most other instances where an encounter with a deceased loved one was described.

9. A check of her medical records reveals that the arrest was mentioned, but not its duration.

10. Only one respondent implied that the illumination hurt his eyes. All others denied that this was the case—usually emphatically.

11. However, it is possible that in this case the individual received an injection of nitrous oxide at the time of his tooth extraction. He himself is not sure and the dentist's records are not available.

12. Two other persons used the same biblical phrase to describe the experience of "a valley."

References

Greyson, Bruce, and Ian Stevenson. 1980. "The Phenomenology of Near-Death Experiences." *American Journal of Psychiatry* 137:1193-96.

Moody, Raymond A., Jr. 1975. *Life After Life*. Atlanta: Mockingbird Books.

_____. 1977. *Reflections on Life After Life*. New York: Bantam Books.

Osis, Karlis, and Erlendur Haraldsson. 1977. *At the Moment of Death*. New York: Avon.

Rawlings, Maurice. 1978. *Beyond Death's Door*. Nashville: Nelson.

Ring, Kenneth. 1980. *Life at Death*. New York: Coward, McCann and Geoghegan.

Sabom, Michael. 1981. *Recollections of Death*. New York: Harper and Row.

_____ and Sarah Kreutziger. 1977. "The Experience of Near Death." *Death Education* 1:195-203.

8

Physicians Evaluate the
Near-Death Experience

Michael B. Sabom and
Sarah S. Kreutziger

RECENTLY, A NEW INTEREST IN THE STUDY of the psychological aspects of death and dying has emerged (Kübler-Ross 1971, 1975). Along with this interest, numerous reports of the unique and detailed experiences of persons encountering near-death situations have appeared in the religious (Graham, 1976; Marshall, 1971; Phillips, 1971), lay (Panati, 1976; Woodward, 1976a; Moody, 1975, Ford, 1971; Leadbeater, 1973), and parapsychological literature (Jacobson, 1974; Thouless, 1972; Osis and Haraldsson, 1962). Over one hundred of these near-death experiences (NDEs) have been reported by Dr. Raymond A. Moody, Jr. in his recent best seller, *Life After Life* (1975). On the jacket of the book, the statement is made that Moody is "convinced that this unexplained phenomenon has great significance for philosophy, medicine, and the ministry, as well as for the way we lead our daily lives." However, little mention of these NDEs has been made in medical publications and few physicians are aware of their occurrence.

Intrigued by the purported nature and significance of these NDEs, we began interviewing survivors of near-fatal encounters in March, 1976 in an effort to document the existence, nature, and clinical implications of the NDE. The results of this twenty month investigation form the basis of this article. Preliminary findings of this study have been reported elsewhere (Sabom and Kreutziger, 1977 a, b, c, d).

One hundred hospital patients (seventy-one male, twenty-nine female) who could clearly recall having suffered a near-fatal crisis resulting in a complete loss of awareness of surroundings (unconsciousness) were interviewed. Sixty-eight of these were obtained from the authors' daily hospital contacts and thirty-two were referred to us from other sources. The mean age of patients at the time of interview was fifty-three years (range seventeen to eighty-six). Psychotic and demented patients were excluded from the study.

Details of the crisis event were obtained from the patient and corroborated by family and referring physician, and medical records when available. When more than one crisis event was recalled, the most recent and/or the one associated with an NDE was selected. Information obtained at the interview included: (1) demographic and sociological data including age, sex, race, years of formal education, occupation, religious affiliation and religiosity; (2) details of the near-death crisis both while conscious and unconscious; and (3) effect of the near-death crisis on the patient's fear of dying and belief in afterlife. Each patient was allowed to describe the experience in his or her own words. If necessary, clarification was later obtained through specific questioning. Religiosity was evaluated using the following scale: 0 for agnostic and 1, 2, 3, 4 for formal religious belief with absent, rare, occasional and weekly church attendance respectively. Knowledge of NDE from other sources was determined at the end of the interview. When possible, interviews were tape recorded for future reference.

Records of each interview were reviewed and the content of each NDE (when present) was analyzed. The sixty-eight patients from our daily rounds, Group A, were then divided into sub-groups with and without recollections of an NDE. Demographic and sociologic data, effects of crisis event on death anxiety and afterlife beliefs, and knowledge of NDE from other sources were statistically compared between these sub-groups. The background characteristics of only these patients were compared, to avoid the biases inherent in comparing demographic and sociologic data in patients referred from different sources. The content of the NDE was analyzed in all patients, however, since this data was felt to be less dependent on the method of patient procurement.

PATIENTS' RECOLLECTIONS

Near-fatal crisis events associated with unconsciousness were found to be as follows: cardiac arrest (67), noncardiac systemic illness (20), accident (5), intraoperative complication (7), and suicide attempt (1). Mean age of patients at time of crisis event was forty-six years (range five to seventy-six).

Thirty-nine of the patients recalled nothing of the period of unconsciousness. Definite recollections while unconscious (NDE) were reported by sixty-one. The details of these sixty-one NDEs were surprisingly consistent and of three types: self-visualization from a position of height (autoscopy—sixteen patients); passage of the consciousness into a foreign region or dimension (transcendence—thirty-two patients); or a combination of autoscopy and transcendence (thirteen patients).

During the autoscopic experience, all patients noted a "floating" sensation "out of the body" unlike any felt before. While "detached" from the physical body, the patient observed his or her own body in clear detail. Nearby objects (many out of "view" of the patient's body) could often be seen (cardiac monitor behind the patient's bed, etc.). In most patients, observation of the type and sequence of resuscitation measures occurred at the time physiologic unconsciousness was most certain (during a grand mal seizure, cardioversion of ventricular fibrillation, injection of intracardiac medications, etc.). In one patient's words, "It was like sitting up in a balcony looking down at a movie." An overwhelming sense of calm and peace pervaded the whole episode. The experience ended abruptly and was followed by the regaining of consciousness.

A typical example of an autoscopic experience is given in the case of a forty-nine-year-old male security guard. Medical records indicate that the patient experienced a cardio-pulmonary arrest while in the hall of the emergency room. Resuscitation attempts were prolonged (approximately thirty minutes). Closed chest massage, artificial respiration with an Ambu bag and other appropriate resuscitation measures were unsuccessful in converting ventricular fibrillation. Respiration and blood pressure were finally restored after two 400 watt-second shocks. An acute anterior myocardial infarction was later diagnosed. The guard recalled his experience in these words:

I just couldn't stand the pain anymore... and then I collapsed. That's when everything went dark and black. After a little while, I was sitting up there somewhere... floating, soft, easy, comfortable, nothing wrong... I could look down, and I had never noticed that the floor was black and white tile, but that's the first thing I remember being conscious of. I recognized myself down there, sort of curled around in a half fetal position. Two or three people lifted me onto a stretcher and strapped my legs and moved me on down the hall. When they first threw me up on the table, the doctor struck me, and I mean he really whacked the hell out of me. He came back with his fist from way behind his head and he hit me right in the center of my chest and then they were pushing on my chest... and they shoved a plastic tube, like you put in an oil can, in my mouth. It was at that point I noticed another table-like arrangement with a bunch of stuff on it. I knew it later to be that machine that they thump you with... [this cart] was making a terrible racket as they were wheeling it down the hall. That caught my attention right away. I could see my right ear and this side of my face because I was looking away. I could hear people talking... it [cardiac monitor] was like an oscilloscope, just a faint white line running across. It wasn't a big scope like they put a TV monitor on you during cardiac cath... It just made the same streak over and over... they put a needle in me, like one of those Aztec Indian rituals where they take the virgin's heart out, they took it two-handed, I thought this very unusual... then they took these round discs with handles on them and put one up here, I think it was larger than the other one, and they put one down here [patient pointed to appropriate positions on chest]... they thumped me and I didn't respond. I thought they had given my body too much voltage. Man, my body jumped about two feet off the table. It appeared to me in some sort of fashion that I had a choice to re-enter my body and take the chances of them bringing me back around or I could just go ahead and die, if I wasn't already dead. I knew I was going to be perfectly safe, whether my body died or not. They thumped me a second time. I re-entered my body just like that. I've lived with this thing for three years and I haven't told anyone because I don't want them to put the straight jacket on me. That was real. It's real as hell. If you want to, you can give me sodium pentothal. It's a pretty kinky experience.

The elements of the transcendent experience were more variable and often colored by personal beliefs and attitudes. One recurrent theme was present, however. The experience usually began with the passage of consciousness into a "black void" or "tunnel." With a sense of being "lifted" or "moved," the patient entered a foreign region or dimension brightly lit and of great beauty. Surroundings were "indescribably beautiful" and usually consisted of trees, grass, flowers, etc. A "border" was sometimes perceived (gate, stream, fence, etc.) over which the patient could not pass. A "brilliant white light" was occasionally present and was thought, by some, to have a religious significance. Deceased relatives, friends, or other people were encountered and a nonverbal interchange of thoughts ensued. The general message of this exchange was perceived by the patient to be that it was "not my time to go" and that "I must return for some reason." Many patients emphatically did not want to "return" because the experience was so enjoyable.

A sixty-seven-year-old housewife suffering from chronic heart failure who became unresponsive in an intensive care unit and had to be cardioverted several times for a "tachycardia" had the following transcendent experience.

> I felt like I was lifted. I don't know how to explain it to you. It was just beautiful... trees were there but they were all in the shadows of gold; no green, no blue, nothing else. It was like a beautiful sunglow and sunset. The water was like a shallow creek... it was like you would go for a splashing wade. All I could hear was the splashing of the water. And on the bank was my grandmother, granddaddy, my mother and daddy, one child that my grandparents had but I knew nothing about, and a man... but I did not see the man... everybody was happy... they didn't say anything. But all that registered with me really and truly was that my husband was coming with outstretched arms in the water and I was coming too. He looked just like when he used to walk into a room... happy... it would have been easy to have gone on with him. I think he would have carried me on across. It seems to me that within a few seconds he would have had a hold of my hand... and within a second or two it all went away, no rhyme or reason. It wasn't my time to go on. It wasn't my decision, because if it had been, I guess I would have [gone]. I don't have any fear of dying...[my doctor] doesn't want me to read that book [Life After Life] for a while. He doesn't want me to be depresseed just yet. But it really hasn't depressed me because I feel like, I'll tell you truthfully, that I'm left here for some reason... what that reason is I'm not going to tell you. I [later] asked my minister "Do you think I'm crazy?"

Thirteen patients experienced both autoscopy and transcendence. The elements of these combined NDEs were similar to those separately outlined above. The following example comes from a fifty-six-year-old executive who had been run over by an automobile with multiple injuries to the head, abdomen, and extremities. While being evaluated in an emergency room, he suffered a cardiac arrest and experienced the following:

When I was in the emergency room I seemed to be there but then I wasn't there. I seemed to see myself on this gurney or whatever and they moved me to a table. I seemed to be one of the participants in there but back further from the table than anyone else...in the background. I was able to look down. I was able to see all this...the table was over at that end of the room and the doctors were on the right side of me and they had a lot of nurses on the left side. There was also a priest there...they didn't have to give me pain shots or anything, because I was completely out of it. I just kept saying, that isn't me...but I knew it was me and that something had happened. I thought the whole thing was strange, I had never experienced anything like it. I wasn't frightened in the least. I was all black from the road tar. I had cuts all over my face that were bleeding. I remember the way the leg was, all the blood; I remember one doctor saying, "He is going to lose his leg." In the meantime they gave me a tourniquet on my leg...the monitor was at the back of my head, in the back of me. I was able to see the line on the monitor...and all of a sudden it stopped and it looked like a TV tube when you reset the tube—you see that green line go across—and it made one continuous noise... then I heard somebody say "It's stopped" or something like that, and I remember one of the doctors banging on my chest, pushing on it. That's when they brought this unit out...they were rubbing those things together, and I was there all this time and I thought, "My God, this can't be me." I came off the table about nine to ten inches. I seemed to arch and then I was in complete, total darkness. I didn't know where I was or what I was doing there or what was happening... time has no bearing on it at all. I started getting scared and all of a sudden there was a light down at the end, the light got brighter, and all of a sudden I seemed to be floating in air, a lot of beautiful blue, the clouds floating by. I was like in a shaft or beam of light and I was traveling through it. Then I had a very gentle pressure on my head, something stopped me and said that I had to go back. And I said, "Why me, Lord?" and whoever it was, said my work wasn't done on earth, that I had to go back. And I felt a great disappointment because it's undescribable what you feel, it's really undescribable, it's so peaceful and restful. I really didn't want to go back. I felt like I could float in there the rest of my life, I mean for all eternity. I started back the way I had come, floating through this light. Before the accident I had always thought that it [dying] would be very unpleasant. I was always frightened of it. Now I'm not afraid any more. I don't talk to anybody [about this]. I'm afraid to because most people think you're sort of batty. [They would say] boy this guy really has got marbles loose up there.

Of the sixty-eight patients in Group A, twenty-nine (43 percent) recalled an NDE. The background characteristics of Group A patients are summarized in Table 1. No significant differences were found between patient groups with and without an NDE except that those recalling an NDE were less frequently aware of similar occurrences from other sources prior to their own experience. Although the reason for this difference is unclear, it decreases the likelihood that subjects with an NDE were merely patterning their experience after the reports of others.

The effects the crisis event had on the death anxieties and afterlife beliefs of Group A patients are summarized in Table 2. The recollection of an NDE was associated with a decrease in death

TABLE 1

Characteristics of Patients in Group A

	With NDE	Without NDE*
Patients	29	39
Age (mean years)	49	52
Sex (male)	23 (79%)	32 (82%)
Race (white)	29 (100%)	35 (90%)
Education (mean years)	11.4	11.0
Occupation		
Professional	2 (7%)	8 (20%)
Clerical, sales	11 (38%)	10 (26%)
Laborer, services	16 (55%)	21 (54%)
Religion		
Christian	25 (86%)	34 (87%)
None	4 (14%)	5 (13%)
Religiosity Index†	2.3	2.3
Other Knowledge of NDE	4 (14%)	25 (64%) (p < .01)

Abbreviation: NDE = near death experience (see text)
*All comparisons between these two groups were not significant at the .05 level unless otherwise noted
†Religiosity index—see text

TABLE 2

Effects of Near-Fatal Encounter on Patients in Group A

	With NDE	Without NDE	With vs. Without
Patients	29	39	
Death Anxiety			
Increased	0	5 (13%)	N.S.
No change	9 (31%)	34 (87%)	p < .001
Decreased	20 (69%)	0	p < .001
Belief in Afterlife			
Increased	20 (69%)	0	p < .001
No change	9 (31%)	39 (100%)	p < .001

Abbreviations: NDE—near death experience (see text);
     N.S.—not significant to .05 level

anxiety and increase in afterlife belief which was significantly different from patients without an NDE (p < .001).

HOW CAN WE EXPLAIN THESE EXPERIENCES?

Knowledge of the NDE is not unique to our time or culture. *The Tibetan Book of the Dead* (Evans-Wentz, 1960) compiled from the teachings of Tibetan sages in the eighth century, A.D. describes a passage similar in many details to the autoscopic and transcendent experiences of our patients. Similar accounts can be found in the literature and arts down through the ages (Heim, 1972; Bierce, 1920; Poe, 1938; Jung, 1961).

We have concluded that the NDE is a real and consistent event for many patients unconscious and near death, and that most patients are reluctant to discuss their experience for fear of ridicule. In addition, we found that the elements of the autoscopic and transcendent experiences of our patients were identical to those reported by Moody, and that . . . sociologic and demographic factors seemingly did not affect the occurrence of NDEs (Table 1).

A generally accepted explanation for these phenomena is not presently available. Several theories have been proposed, including:

(1) A "mental picture" of ongoing events could conceivably be constructed solely from verbal input into the brain of a semiconscious patient. However, some of our patients gave detailed autoscopic accounts of themselves and their surroundings from a

time when no one else was present. In others, the recalled details included visual descriptions of objects (including size, shape, location and usage), and events not ordinarily discussed during a resuscitation attempt (i.e., oral airway, defibrillator paddles, intracardiac needle, etc.).

(2) A temporal lobe seizure resulting from brain hypoxia could cause visual illusions and feelings of unreality in patients near death. However, this seizure disorder also produces: (a) illusions of people as distorted, flattened, or half-figures; (b) sudden feelings of despair, guilt, anxiety, and terror; (c) suicidal and aggressive urges; and (d) vestibular and olfactory experiences (Slater and Roth, 1969). None of our patients reported these sensations. In addition, the accurate visual description of ongoing events which occur during unconsciousness could not be easily explained by the seizure hypothesis.

(3) Drugs can produce vivid and convincing distortions of reality. However, the medical records of several of our patients indicated no drug usage at the time of unconsciousness. In addition, the wide variety of positive and negative experiences reported by individuals during drug-related hallucinations (Melges, Tinklenberg, Hillister, et al., 1970) does not jibe with the consistency of the elements in NDEs. When a patient with an NDE had previously had a delusional experience from medicinal narcotics, this drug-related hallucination was perceived to be clearly different from the NDE (the NDE being clearer, not distorted, more "real," and associated with a calm and peace not previously encountered).

(4) A form of "depersonalization" has been described in persons faced with extreme danger (Noyes and Kletti, 1976 a,b). Many of the subjective phenomena attributed to "depersonalization" (increased speed of thoughts, automatic movements, lack of emotion), however, were not reported by our patients. In addition, the depersonalization hypothesis is based on a study of individuals who had perceived the threat of extreme danger, but had rarely experienced unconsciousness or had been physically near death. Many of our patients, however, suffered unconsciousness and physical near-death without prior warning (Stokes-Adams attacks, cardiac arrest, etc.).

(5) Autoscopic hallucinations have been described in psychiatric patients, and consist of seeing a "double" which usually appears

suddenly and without warning (Lukianowicz, 1958). However, during these hallucinations, the perception is *of* the "double" *by* the physical body ("original"). This "double" is most frequently seen only as a face or face and bust, is usually transparent and commonly imitates the movements and facial expression of its "original." The emotional reaction to seeing one's "double" is often sadness accompanied by a feeling of coldness and weariness. These features of autoscopic hallucinations are clearly different from those found in NDEs.

(6) Spiritualists have long maintained that the physical body can make "contact" with another dimension through "astral projection" (Leadbeater, 1973). In addition, religious writings have long alluded to the promise of an afterlife. A discussion of the relationship of these hypotheses to NDEs falls outside the purview of this paper.

Although these NDEs are presently inexplicable, their effect on the death anxieties of the individuals involved was often dramatic (Table 2). Most of our patients emphasized that their previous fears of death were definitely reduced, if not totally eliminated, by the NDE. Alleviation of this fear, in turn, assisted many in coping with the day-to-day uncertainties of a terminal condition. In addition, the patient who had experienced a near-death phenomenon was often relieved at being able to discuss his experience in an atmosphere of openness and understanding and was comforted by the knowledge that others had had similar encounters. Finally, medical and paramedical personnel involved in patient care have indicated that an awareness of these NDE (from local presentations) has been meaningful in both their personal and professional lives (unpublished data).

In summary, sixty-one NDEs were found in interviews of one hundred patients who had been unconscious and near death. While unconscious, sixteen patients viewed their body and physical surroundings from a detached position of height several feet above the ground (autoscopy), thirty-one experienced the passage of consciousness into a foreign region or dimension (transcendence), and thirteen experienced both autoscopy and transcendence. Social and demographic characteristics of patients, or knowledge of NDEs from other sources, seemingly did not affect the occurrence of an NDE. Patients recalling an NDE emphasized that their previous fears of death were definitely reduced, if not totally eliminated, by the event. The NDE cannot be adequately explained at the present time. Further investigation into the cause of NDEs and the implications these experiences may have on personal and social concepts of death and dying is needed.

References

Bierce, A. 1920. "An Occurrence at Owl Creek Bridge." *The Great Modern American Stories.* New York: Boni and Liveright.

Evans-Wentz, W.Y. (ed.) 1960. *The Tibetan Book of the Dead.* New York: Oxford University Press.

Ford, A. 1971. *The Life Beyond Death.* New York: Putnam.

Graham, B. 1976. *Angels: God's Secret Agents.* New York: Guideposts Associates.

Heim, A. 1892. "Remarks on Fatal Falls." *Yearbook of the Swiss Alpine Club,* *27*:327-37. (Trans. by R. Noyes and R. Kletti in *Omega, 3*:45-52, 1972.)

Jacobson, N.O. 1974. *Life Without Death?* New York: Dell.

Jung, C.G. 1961. *Memories, Dreams, Reflections.* New York: Pantheon.

Kübler-Ross, E. 1971. *On Death and Dying.* New York: Macmillan Company.

———. 1975. *Death: The Final Stage of Growth.* New Jersey: Prentice-Hall, Inc.

Leadbeater, C.W. 1973. *The Astral Plane.* India: Theosophical Publishing House.

Lukianowicz, N. 1958. "Autoscopic Phenomena" *Archives of Neurology and Psychiatry, 80*:199-220.

Marshall, C. 1971. *A Man Called Peter.* New York: Avon.

Melges, F.T., Tinklenberg, J.R., Hollister, L.E., et al. 1970. "Temporal Disintegration and Depersonalization During Marihuana Intoxication." *Archives of General Psychiatry, 23*:294-310.

Moody, R.A. 1975. *Life After Life.* Covington, GA: Mockingbird Books.

Noyes, R., Jr., and Kletti, R. 1976a. "Depersonalization in the Face of Life Threatening Danger: A Description." *Psychiatry, 39*:19-27.

———. 1976b. "Depersonalization in the Face of Life Threatening Danger: An Interpretation." *Omega, 7*:103-14.

Osis, K., and Haraldsson, E. 1962. *Deathbed Observations by Physicians and Nurses: A Cross-cultural Survey.* New York: Parapsychology Foundation.

Panati, C. 1976. "Is There Life After Death?" *Family Circle, 89:*78, 84, 90.

Phillips, J.B. 1971. *Your God is Too Small.* New York: Macmillan.

Poe, E.A. 1938. "A Descent into the Maelstrom." *The Complete Tales and Poems of Edgar Allen Poe.* New York: Modern Library.

Sabom, M.B., and Kreutziger, S. 1977a. "The Experience of Near-Death." *Death Education, 1:*195-203.

_____. 1977b. "Near-death Experiences." *Journal of the Florida Medical Association, 64:*648-50.

_____. 1977c. Near-death Experiences letter. *New England Journal of Medicine, 297:*1071.

_____. 1977d. Insight into the Process of Death letter. *Psychology Today, 10:*7.

Slater, E., and Roth, M. 1969. *Clinical Psychiatry.* Baltimore: Williams and Wilkins Company.

Thouless, R.H. 1972. *From Anecdote to Experiment in Psychical Research.* London: Routledge and Kegan.

Woodward, K.L. 1976a. "There Is Life After Death." *McCall's 103:*134-39.

Woodward, K.L. 1976b. "Life After Death." *Newsweek, 41:*July 12.

9

The Dying Patient's Concern with Life After Death

Charles A. Garfield

I BELIEVE IT IS POSSIBLE THAT REALISTIC acceptance of death is for some individuals intimately related to near-death consciousness-altering experiences of a transcendent nature (Garfield 1977b). About 21 percent of the terminally ill patients I have interviewed had such experiences in the preterminal and/or terminal phases of their illness. Their general reluctance to report these perceptions was directly related to a fear either of being labeled insane or of having their experiences disqualified as hallucinatory. An increased understanding of the dying process, of intense psychic transformation, may require us to acknowledge, along with Laing, that the

> ego is the instrument for living in this world. If the ego is fragmented or destroyed (by the insurmountable contradictions of certain situations, by toxins, by chemical changes, etc.), the person experiencing this transformation may be exposed to other worlds, as "real" but different from the more familiar territory of dreams, imagination, perception, and fantasy. [Laing, 1972]

The near-death experiences recorded in the medical and psychological literature are not positive proof of life after death; rather they are altered-state experiences not at all specific to the dying process. I have received several letters from women who had very similar experiences during natural childbirth. I believe the near-death experiences described in this book are a subclass of a larger group of altered-state experiences attainable through a variety of techniques and circumstances.

In the past three years, I have worked with 215 cancer patients who subsequently died. I spent an average of three to four hours a week with them for a period ranging from several weeks to almost two years. Among the 22 percent who told me of their altered state experiences, four groups emerged.

1. One experienced a powerful white light and celestial music (as in Moody's accounts) as well as an encounter (similar to that reported by Osis and Haraldsson) with a religious figure or deceased relative. The patients described these as "incredibly real, peaceful and beautiful."

2. A second experienced demonic figures, nightmarish images of great lucidity.

3. A third reported dreamlike images, sometimes "blissful," sometimes "terrifying," sometimes alternating. The images were not nearly as lucid as those related by the first two groups. However, they appeared to have as great a variation in content.

4. The final groups experienced the Void or a tunnel or both. That is, the patients reported drifting endlessly in outer space or being encapsulated in a limited environment with obvious spatial constraints. A common theme in their accounts was the contrast between maximal freedom and maximal constraint with, in some cases, fluctuation from one to the other.

My work has included interviews with individuals who have had near-death experiences or who have been pronounced clinically dead and then revived. In an effort to evaluate the anecdotal reports of Moody and Kübler-Ross, I conducted in-depth interviews with thirty-six intensive care or coronary care patients. Since my primary function is to provide basic emotional support, I was often the first person to interact with the patient for an appreciable length of time following his brush with death. My contact occurred anywhere from three hours to two days following the incident. Eighteen patients reported no memory of the event at all. Their last memory before losing consciousness was of being in their hospital room and when they awoke they were either in the ICU or CCU "hooked up to the hardware." Seven reported experiences similar to those collected by Moody, Kübler-Ross, and Osis, including seeing a bright light, hearing "celestial" music, and meeting religious figures or deceased relatives. Four reported lucid visions of a demonic or nightmarish nature. Four reported having dreamlike images; in two instances entirely positive and the other two alternating between positive and negative. Three patients reported drifting endlessly in outer space among the planets, but loose as if thrown from a space ship. No significant changes in content were expressed by any of the patients in three interviews conducted at weekly intervals following the event.

In light of this research, three main observations seem important.

1. It appears that not everyone dies a blissful, accepting death. My friend's tortuous, labored breathing during the twenty-four hours before she died hardly appeared blissful. I hope those who suggest that she was really "feeling no pain" thanks to the "immunity" provided by her comatose state or because she was really "out of her body" are correct. However, almost as many of the dying patients I interviewed reported negative visions (encounters with demonic figures, and so forth) as reported blissful experiences, while some reported both.

2. Pelletier and Garfield (1976) note that context is a powerful variable in such altered state experiences as the hypnotic, meditative, psychedelic, schizophrenic. In keeping with the early LSD research, we might very well find that a caring environment including supportive family, friends, and staff is an important factor in maximizing the likelihood of a positive altered state experience for the dying. Certainly, helping dying patients relate to their experiences in a constructive fashion rather than imposing psychiatric judgment is the more supportive stance. Whatever they represent, those experiences were very important to the dying patients who had them. We need to examine more carefully the impact of context on the dying process. Context includes the quality of advocacy and nonjudgmental caring offered by family and staff. Contextual as well as psychobiological factors may significantly influence the altered state experiences of the dying patient. We may discover that we are dealing not only with the "fact of communication with the dead," whether literal or not, but also with the issue of how we and our patients relate to those experiences. We would do well to remember that when Goethe was about to die he cried, "Light, light, the world needs more light." It was many years later that Unamuno responded, "Goethe was wrong; what he should

have said was 'Warmth, the world needs more warmth.' We shall not die from the darkness, but from the cold."

3. Robert Kastenbaum (1977) notes that "the happily, happily theme threatens to draw attention away from the actual situations of the dying person, their loved ones and their care givers over the days, weeks, and months preceding death. What happens up to the point of that fabulous transition from life to death recedes into the background. This could not be more unfortunate." Will our aversion to death take yet another form and leave us prey to promises of life after death which we cannot integrate emotionally? It is certainly feasible that we run the risk of once again denying death and perhaps biasing our level of care to those who are dying. Will our "knowledge of life after death" leave us in a position to "abandon life-saving efforts for some people, try less hard to save lives at critical moments" (Kastenbaum, 1977)?

> It is hard to have patience with people who say "There is no death" or "Death doesn't matter." There is death, and whatever happens has consequences, and it and they are irrevocable and irreversible. You might as well say that birth doesn't matter. I look up at the night sky. Is anything more certain than that in all those vast times and spaces, if I were allowed to search them, I should nowhere find her face, her voice, her touch? She died. She is dead. Is the word so difficult to learn? [Lewis, 1961]

C.S. Lewis astutely observes that whether we view death as annihilation or transition, it is a real and often monumental event. An emotional blow associated with a change of form. Those I love in the form I love no longer exist. Those having near-death experiences exuberantly extol the virtues of loving and caring for one's fellow man. So let us have the courage to realize that death often will be a bitter pill to swallow. Our pain will almost always accompany the deaths of those we most love. Our wish will almost always be that help and caring are available.

References

Garfield, C. 1977. *Rediscovery of the Body: A Psychosomatic View of Life and Death.* New York: Dell.

Kastenbaum, R. 1977. "Temptations from the Ever After," *Human Behavior,* 6:28-33.

Laing, R. 1972. "Transcendental Experience." In *The Highest State of Consciousness*, ed. John White. New York: Anchor.

Lewis, C.S. 1961. *A Grief Observed*. New York: Seabury.

Pelletier, K., and C. Garfield. 1976. *Consciousness: East and West*. New York: Harper and Row.

10

Near-Death Experiences
of Mormons

Craig R. Lundahl

INTRODUCTION

IN THE PAST FEW YEARS THERE HAS been considerable interest in the events occuring during near-death encounters. This interest has been stimulated primarily by the widely publicized research on death and on near death by Elisabeth Kübler-Ross (1969) and Raymond A. Moody, Jr. (1975) and their respective best sellers, *On Death and Dying* and *Life After Life.*

Several recent studies have focused on near-death experiences. Moody reported on 150 cases of persons who experienced an apparent clinical death or who experienced, in the course of an accident, severe injury, or illness, a very close brush with death. Based on his study, Moody was able to develop a list of common elements of near-death experiences. Noyes and Kletti (1976) gave a descriptive analysis of 114 accounts of near-death experiences obtained from 104 persons. They found remarkably similar descriptions to those given in Moody's study. Sabom and Kreutziger (1977) interviewed fifty patients with documented near-fatal encounters. Again the findings reported by these investigators were consistent

---

"Near-Death Experiences of Mormons" by Craig R. Lundahl, selected portions of a paper presented at the 1979 American Psychological Association Annual Convention at New York City and portions published in *Free Inquiry in Creative Sociology*, 7, No. 2 (November, 1979): 101-4, 107. Copyright © 1979 by the Oklahoma Sociological Association. Reprinted by permission of the publisher and the author.

with the findings of earlier investigators. In 1977, Osis and Haraldsson reported on deathbed observations in the United States and in India. In their study, physicians and nurses completed questionnaires and were subsequently interviewed concerning 442 cases in the United States and 435 cases in India. They found that four-fifths of the apparitions appearing to terminal patients portrayed deceased persons and religious figures and that three out of four apparitions were experienced as having come to take patients away to a postmortem existence.

The purpose of this paper is to provide further research on the subject of near-death experiences by reporting on a limited number of cases of the near-death experiences of members of a particular religious group, the Church of Jesus Christ of Latter-day Saints, more commonly known as Mormons, and to compare these near-death experiences to those reports by other researchers.

Although accounts of near-death experiences have circulated among Mormons for many years, only one study has reported anything on the subject. Ray R. Canning (1965) reported on the near-death experiences of seven Mormons who had died and returned to life. Canning found that most of his subjects reported a displacement of the conscious self from the physical body and saw their physical bodies lying in death. Some of the subjects experienced travel through time and space and all except one left their earthly environment after their death or near-death experience. Two of the subjects reported that guardian angels or guides were present to lead them. Several of the subjects noted the vegetation, landscape, and buildings in the afterworld as well as the orderliness and pleasant busyness there. Several subjects described conversations with friends or relatives who had died. One respondent noted that the dead did not appear to be at the same age as they were at the time of their death. Two reports indicate that the members of the spirit world are dressed variously but usually in white. Several subjects resisted returning to life. Of the five respondents who described the sensations of returning to life, only one experienced considerable pain.

The uncommon number of written historical descriptions of near-death experiences as well as the openly expressed accounts of near-death experiences among Mormons today is probably explainable because of the social values found among Latter-day Saints. In his well-known study, *The Mormons,* O'Dea pointed out that

Mormons have a definite belief in an afterlife (1957, p. 130). Their social value system is supportive of and encourages the exchange of near-death experiences among the membership in church meetings and on other occasions to a much greater extent than would be found among most other groups. Moody (1975, p. 85) found in his study, as have other researchers, that although persons having near-death experiences were certain of the reality and importance of what happened to them, they also realized

> that our contemporary society is just not the sort of environment in which reports of this nature would be received with sympathy and understanding. Indeed, many have remarked that they realized from the very beginning that others would think they were mentally unstable if they were to relate their experiences. So, they have resolved to remain silent on the subject or else to reveal their experiences only to some very close relative.

METHODS

This study is based on eleven nonrandom accounts of near-death experience by Mormons between the years of 1838 and 1976. The study is limited to accounts of individuals who were adjudged dead or who experienced a very close brush with death in the course of an accident, a severe injury, or an illness. Of the two accounts obtained through interviews, both experienced close brushes with death in the course of an accident and severe injury.

Two methods were used to collect the information for the study. The method used for the collection of information on nine of the accounts was the analysis of secondary sources of data. The method used for collection of information on the other two accounts was the free story interview.

The accounts of near-death experiences in this study may not be representative of all Mormon near-death experiences between 1838 and 1976 because of the low number of accounts, their nonrandom selection, and the subjective reporting of the accounts.

CASES

Probably one of the earliest recorded Mormon accounts of a near-death experience was that of a Latter-day Saint woman in 1838 who related her experience to her husband afterwards, which he described as follows.

Her spirit left her body, and she saw it lying upon the bed and the sisters there weeping. She looked at them and at me, and upon her babe, and, while gazing upon the scene, two persons came into the room carrying a coffin and told her they had come for her body. One of these messengers informed her that she could have her choice: she might go to rest in the spirit world, or, on one condition, she could have the privilege of returning to her tabernacle and continuing her labors upon the earth. The condition was, that if she felt that she could stand by her husband, and with him pass through all the cares, trials, tribulation and afflictions of life which he would be called to pass through for the gospel's sake unto the end. When she looked at the situation of her husband and child she said: "Yes, I will do it." [Woodruff, 1909, pp. 59-60]

In 1852, a sixteen-year-old Latter-day Saint journeyed into the spirit world. She wrote that her mother escorted her on a visit of the spirit world. During her journey, she reported seeing an unfinished building in the spirit world. She was led by her mother into a very large and beautiful bedroom in the building where she saw a young boy who had been buried on the plains and some other persons she recognized. While in the building, she looked in another room and saw the prophet Joseph Smith, founder of the Mormon Church, who was walking up and down the room with his head bowed as though in thought, as well as several other men, who were writing. During her visit, she was told by her mother that her mother's dress had been given to her by the Lord and that her mother took her turn working in the kitchen (Crowther, 1967, p. 382).

In 1856, a Latter-day Saint man who was near death told of two visits to the spirit world. In these informative near-death experiences, reported by a close friend, the man told of an order, government, buildings, and gardens in the spirit world, and his dislike to return and resume his body.

When in the spirit world, I saw the order of righteous men and women; beheld them organized in their several grades, and there appeared to be no obstruction to my vision; I could see every man and woman in their grade and order. I looked to see whether there was any disorder there, but there was none; neither could I see any death nor any darkness, disorder or confusion. He said that the people he there saw were organized in family capacities; and when he looked at them he saw grade after grade and all were organized and in perfect harmony....

He saw the righteous gathered together in the spirit world, and there were no wicked spirits among them. He saw his wife; she was the first person that came to him. He saw many that he knew, but did not have conversation with any except his wife, Caroline. She came to him, and he said that she looked beautiful and had their little child, that died on the Plains, in her arms....

"To my astonishment," he said, "when I looked at families there was a deficiency in some, there was a lack, for I saw families that would not be permitted to come and dwell together, because they had not honored their calling here...."

He also spoke of the buildings he saw there, remarking that the Lord gave Solomon wisdom and poured gold and silver into his hands that he might display his skill and ability, and said that the temple erected by Solomon was much inferior to the most ordinary buildings he saw in the spirit world....

In regard to gardens, says Brother Grant, "I have seen good gardens on this earth, but I never saw any to compare with those that were there. I saw flowers of numerous kinds, and some with from fifty to a hundred different colored flowers growing upon one stalk...."

After mentioning the things that he had seen, he spoke of how much he disliked to return and resume his body, after having seen the beauty and glory of the spirit world.

After speaking of the gardens and the beauty of everything there, Brother Grant said that he felt extremely sorrowful at having to leave so beautiful a place and come back to earth, for he looked upon his body with loathing, but was obliged to enter it again.... [Lundwall, p. 71-73]

In Grant's account, he also mentioned he had seen a realm occupied by evil spirits.

In the early 1860s a Latter-day Saint was badly injured in an accident and related:

His spirit left his body and stood, as it were, in the air above it. He could see his body and the men standing around and he heard their conversation. At his option he could re-enter his body or remain in spirit. His reflection upon his responsibility to his family and his great desire to live caused him to choose to enter his body again and live. As he did so he regained consciousness and experienced severe pains incident to the injuries which he had suffered from the accident. [Hinckley 1959, p. 183]

In 1891, a Latter-day Saint who was a girl of fifteen suffering from scarlet fever reported having a near-death experience. She said her spirit left her body, and it took her some time to make up her mind to leave because she could hear and see her folks crying and mourning over her death. She said that as soon as she had a glimpse of the other world she was anxious to go; that all her cares and worries left her. She could hear the most delightful music and singing that she had ever heard. She reported entering a large hall that was so long that she could not see the end of it. It was filled with people, including a great many relatives and friends. She said she visited with many of them and noticed that everybody appeared to be perfectly happy. Some of the persons she visited with inquired about their friends and relatives on the earth. She noted that all but one person was dressed in white or cream. As she reached the end of the long room, she opened another door and went into a room filled with children. She reported that the children were arranged in a perfect order according to age and size and seemed to be convened in a Primary or Sunday School.

It was while she was listening to the children sing that she was told, "You must come back as your mission is not yet finished here on earth." As she returned through the large room, she told the people she was going back to the earth. They seemed to want her to stay with them. She obeyed the call even though she did not want to leave this beautiful place where perfect peace and happiness prevailed and where there was no suffering and no sorrow. As she returned she could see her body lying on the bed and the folks gathered about in the room. She hesitated for a moment, then thought, "Yes, I will go back for a little while." She reported there was practically no pain on leaving the body in death but there was intense pain, almost unbearable, in coming back to life. Afterward, she related her experience to some close relatives. After she described the appearance of unrecognizable persons in the long room, many were identified by her relatives as aunts and second cousins who had died before she was born (Snow, 1929, p. 973-74).

In 1898, a Mormon missionary who was stricken with malaria, reported this near-death experience:

> My spirit left the body; just how I cannot tell. But I perceived myself standing some four or five feet in the air, and saw my body lying on the bed. I felt perfectly natural, but as this was a new condition I began to make observations. I turned my head, shrugged my shoulders, felt with my hands, and realized that it was I myself. I also knew that my body was lying lifeless, on the bed. While I was in a new environment, it did not seem strange, for I realized everything that was going on, and perceived that I was the same in the spirit as I had

been in the body. While contemplating this new condition, something attracted my attention, and on turning around I beheld a personage, who said: "You did not know that I was here." I replied: "No, but I see you are. Who are you?" "I am your guardian angel; I have been following you constantly while on earth." I asked: "What will you do now?" He replied: "I am to report your presence, and you will remain here until I return."

The guardian angel returned to inform the missionary that his eldest sister, who had died earlier, would come for a visit shortly. Thereafter, his sister and then other deceased relatives arrived. After some time was spent in conversation, the guide returned to take the missionary to a group of apostles where he was asked several times if he wanted to remain in the spirit world. He replied every time that he was satisfied in the spirit world. After an inquiry of why he was asked so often if he desired to remain, the missionary was informed that his progenitors had made a request that if he chose to return to the earth that he might be granted this privilege of returning. At this point of indecision by the missionary, he was allowed to see what would take place if he remained in the spirit world. He was able to see, among other things, the messages sent concerning his death, the preparations made for the shipment of his body to Utah, and the reactions of his relatives to his death. He decided to return after seeing his father's great anguish over his death. He stated that he did not know how his spirit entered the body. After he entered his body he saw no more of the messengers who had been accompanying him, but he did have vivid recollections of all that had taken place (Johnson, 1920, pp. 451-53).

In 1914, another Latter-day Saint woman related a near-death experience. She had been experiencing considerable sickness due to an infected hand and had contracted a severe cold, which settled in her lungs and caused her to be near death. About midday, she noticed a soft, bright light in her room. Immediately after the light appeared, so did her dead parents and some other dead relatives. During the several hours which followed, they talked about the reason one particular relative had died leaving behind her small children and about some religious matters. She was also directed to do ordinance work for her dead kindred. During this visitation, she stated that her father was dressed in his military uniform, whereas the other visitors were attired in ordinary clothing. She also stated that during the visitation her son, who was in the adjoining room, came into the room several times to inquire if she needed anything. While her son was in the room her visitors would retire and then reappear when he was gone so that the conversation could continue. As the visitation closed and the visitors began to depart, her father said he would come to her that evening. She reported that he did indeed return for her as she slept and that they went to an area where a large congregation of people were shut up within walls. She was introduced to this large group by her father who said that she had agreed earlier that day to attend to their temple ordinances. When she awoke in the morning, her sickness had disappeared as she was promised the day before. She said later that the more she did to complete the ordinance work which she was instructed to do by her father, the better was the condition of her hand (Wilson, 1915).

A Latter-day Saint who was crushed by a hay derrick reported:

> My spirit left the body, and I could see it lying under the derrick, and at that moment my guardian angel, my mother, and my sister Ann were beside me. My mother died January 31, 1918, and my sister at the age of four years. I saw that her spirit was full grown in stature and also seemed very intelligent.

This person also recorded that he was introduced to the heads of five generations of his father's people and that he was shown the spirits of the children that would yet come to his family if he were faithful. He pointed out that they were full grown but in a different sphere than those who had lived on the earth. He was also instructed on religious matters and met with his two brothers-in-law who were laboring in missionary work. Before his return, he was also requested to perform ordinance work for persons he knew previously on the earth (Crowther, 1967, p. 392).

A Mormon who died of a strangulated hernia in 1923 and then returned to life reported the following:

> Suddenly, I was stricken with a coldness that attacked my feet and hands. It moved up my limbs and up my arms towards my body. I felt it reach my heart. There was a slight murmur. I gasped for breath and lapsed into unconsciousness, so far as all things mortal were concerned. Then I awoke in full possession of all my faculties in another sphere of life. I stood apart from my body and looked at it. I saw it lying upon the bed. I noticed that its eyes were partly closed and that the chin had dropped. I was now without pain, and the joy of freedom I felt and the peace of mind that came over me were the

sweetest sensations I had ever experienced in all my life. I lost all sense of time and space. The law of gravitation had no hold upon me.

He turned to see his little daughter who died many years earlier.

She was more mature than when she passed away, having the intelligence of an adult, and was most beautiful to my eyes, so full of life and so intelligent and sweet. As she came towards me she raised her right hand and said, "Go back, papa, I want Richard first. Then grandma must come, and then mama is coming, before you."

The next thing I knew was my body gasping for breath. I felt my heart action start and I was conscious of the coldness leaving my body just as it had come. All numbness left me and the natural warmth returned. I felt the nurse shaking me and heard her say, "Mr. Monson, you must not let yourself slip like that again."

He later reported that his family members passed away in the exact order outlined by his deceased daughter (Stokes, 1945, pp. 78-79).

In 1972, a young Latter-day Saint woman was severely injured in a serious accident. Immediately following the accident, she remembered that she felt like her body was falling off a bed or descending or falling down a tunnel that seemed to be somewhat similar to a dark staircase. She said,

As I reached the end of the tunnel, I felt an urge to turn back, but I recall I couldn't stop the falling or drifting sensation and I couldn't force my body to turn around. I remember seeing instances of my life that had occurred in the past but they only took seconds to relate. But I remember details, conversations, and they were exactly like they had occurred in the past. The incidences were filled with interactions of loved ones and conversations and memories of my life up to that point. After the flashback, I recall thinking to myself, "I'm dying, I think this is the end." I felt my body or my spirit rise and observed myself pinned under the car. I was actually watching myself. I distinctly remember watching others at the scene of the accident observe myself and I remember looking at my own self from another person's perspective. I remember going back to the stairway and seeing a beam of light at the top. I wanted to go back to the light and I fell back asleep.

After her recovery, this woman told her husband who sustained only minor injuries in the accident with her, what happened at the accident scene. He was totally amazed at her accurate and detailed description of the events surrounding the accident while she was unconscious (Lundahl, 1976).

In 1976, another young Latter-day Saint woman was seriously injured in an automobile accident. Almost immediately, she found herself walking up a steep incline where she passed a large number of people. Finally she came to a woman dressed in white who told her she must return to her body and that an ambulance was coming for her. She told the woman that she "had died and that it was a little late for an ambulance." She was told that she had more to do and more instructions would be given to her later, and again, she was told to return to her body. As she went back down the incline, she saw her body on the ground by her car and all the people standing around. She said that "the people were taking care of her, taking care of her immediate needs, and doctoring her head." Then her spirit entered her body and she became conscious (Lundahl, 1977).

DISCUSSION

The data from the Mormon accounts of near-death experiences suggest that certain events or elements are particularly prevalent during these near-death experiences. These events include the movement by the subject out of the physical body, the meeting of others whether it be close relatives, friends, or a guardian angel, the movement of the subject from his earthly environments into another sphere or world and coming-back to this world experiences.

When the near-death experiences described in this study are compared to those of Moody, Noyes and Kletti, and Sabom and Kreutziger, we find that many of the events are remarkably similar. It is particularly interesting that the results of this study are so alike considering the fact that several of the Mormon accounts of near-death experience are more than a century old.

A comparison of the results of this study to those earlier studies show that all or eleven of the Mormon subjects experienced Noyes and Kletti's subjective phenomena of detachment from the body and that nine experienced some control by an external force (see Table 1).

All of the Mormon subjects experienced Moody's common element of being "out of the body," nine experienced Moody's common element of "meeting others" and nine had experiences related to coming back. Six experienced Moody's common element of "cities of light" (1977, pp. 15-18). Under this common element

TABLE 1

A Placement of Eleven Mormon Accounts of Near-Death Experiences According to Events During Near-Death Experiences Used by Noyes and Kletti, Moody, and Sabom and Kreutziger*

Noyes and Kletti's Subjective Phenomena During Extreme Danger	Event Frequency of Mormon Accounts	Moody's Common Elements During a Near-Death Experience	Event Frequency of Mormon Accounts	Sabom and Kreutziger's Experience Types	Event Frequency of Mormon Accounts
Altered passage of time	1	Ineffability	0	Autoscopy	7
Unusually vivid thoughts	1	Hearing the news	1	Transcendence	6
Sense of harmony or unity	2	Feelings of peace and quiet	2		
Increased speed of thoughts	0	The noise	0		
Sense of detachment	0	The dark tunnel	1		
Detachment from body	11	Out of the body	11		
Feeling of unreality	0	Meeting others	9		
Automatic movements	1	The being of light	1		
Revival of memories	1	The review	1		
Lack of emotion	0	The border or limit	0		
Great understanding	0	Vision of knowledge	0		
Sharper vision or hearing	1	Cities of light	6		
Colors or visions	0	A realm of bewildered spirits	2		
Control of external force	9	Supernatural rescues	1		
Objects small or far away	0	Coming back	9		
Vivid mental images	1				
Voices, music, or sounds	1				

*The categories are from Russell Noyes and Roy Kletti, "Depersonalization in the Face of Life-Threatening Danger: A Description," *Psychiatry*, 39 (1976):19-27; Raymond A. Moody, *Life After Life* (Covington, Georgia: Mockingbird Books, 1975), pp. 25-84; Raymond A. Moody, *Reflections on Life After Life* (Covington, Georgia: Mockingbird Books, 1977), pp. 9-28; and M.B. Sabom and S. Kreutziger, "The Experience of Near-Death," *Death Education*, 1 (1977):195-203.

was placed any Mormon subject who saw buildings or entered rooms or appeared to have visited in a community in the so-called "other world."

The type of experiences of the subjects studied by Sabom and Kreutziger were classified as either autoscopic experiences or transcendental experiences or both. They defined autoscopy as denoting self-visualization from a detached position of height and transcendence as denoting passage of the consciousness into a foreign region or dimension. Table 1 shows that seven of the Mormon subjects experienced autoscopy while six experienced transcendence.

A comparison of the results of this study to those of Canning's study of seven cases of Mormon near-death experiences shows that the results of both studies are very similar. Canning found that most of his subjects reported a displacement of the conscious self from the physical body and saw their body lying in death as did nine of the subjects in this study. All but one of Canning's subjects reported leaving their earthly environment after death or near death as did six of the subjects in this study. Several of Canning's Mormon subjects noted vegetation, landscape, and buildings in the after-world as well as an orderliness and pleasant busyness and other conditions there, as did four of the subjects in this study. Several of Canning's subjects also described conversations with deceased friends or relatives, as did seven of the subjects of this study.

Some of the finer details occurring during near-death experiences used by Moody and Noyes and Kletti, such as "the dark tunnel," "the review," "revival of memories," and "vivid mental images," were not described by any of the historical accounts of the Mormons, but may have occurred. Nevertheless, some of these details were mentioned by a Mormon subject who experienced a recent near-death experience. This discrepancy may be due to the fact that in earlier periods Mormons who had near-death experiences were inclined to give written descriptions of larger events rather than the finer details of their experiences.

Among the Mormon subjects, there was a tendency to describe their near-death experiences in terminology familiar to their subcultural group and to describe various social phenomena in terms of their own cultural conditioning. For example, there was a tendency among those who entered the other world to observe particular activities such as organizational arrangements and family structure. Mormons are exposed to certain organizational and family structures in their church activities and their daily lives and would initially observe similar structures in a new environment. In other words, the observer sees what he is trained to see.

The data are not conclusive on the length of time of these Mormon near-death encounters since most of the accounts are of a historical nature. It does appear that several of the Mormon subjects may have experienced what Moody calls near-death encounters of an extreme duration (1977, p. 9). An unusually high percentage of the Mormon subjects did enter into another sphere or world. Moody later found this element far less common than in his original eleven elements and that this unusual element occurred exclusively in the reports of subjects who had near-death encounters of extreme duration. The unusually high incidence of Mormon subjects who enter another sphere or world may be due to nonrandom selection of the accounts, to the greater likelihood of Mormons encountering in-depth, near-death experiences writing about them than those who did not have such experiences, or to earlier cases in which persons experienced near-death encounters of an extreme nature without the intervention of modern medical technologies. With modern medical assistance, near-death encounters of most persons can be expected to be of short duration. Thus, it appears reasonable that the large majority of present-day cases of near-death experiences will not include the less-common elements of the "vision of knowledge," "cities of light," and a "realm of bewildered spirits" as identified by Moody (1977, pp. 9-22). More importantly, the Mormon accounts do give us a greater insight into the activities and structures of the "other world" which has yet to be described in detail.

Finally, it was quite common to find two other infrequently mentioned events occurring during the near-death experiences of the Mormon subjects. Those events include: (1) requests to do something in this world from those in the other world and (2) the reception of religious and other types of instruction from those in the other world.

SUMMARY

This paper describes the accounts of near-death experiences of Mormons occurring between the years of 1838 and 1976. The findings suggest that certain events are particularly prevalent during the near-death experiences of the subjects. These events are: (1) the movement by the subject out of the physical body, (2) meeting others, such as close relatives, friends, or guardian angels, (3) the movement of the subject from the earthly environment into another sphere or world, and (4) coming back to this world experiences. When the findings of this study are compared to those of other researchers, they are found to be very similar even though several of the Mormon accounts are over a century old. Many of the Mormon subjects appear to have experienced near-death encounters of an extreme duration since a high percentage of them entered into another sphere or world. More importantly, the Mormon accounts give us a greater insight into the activities and structures of the perceived "other world." Common events occurring during the near-death experiences of the Mormon subjects which are not expressly listed elements or events in the work of other researchers are requests to do something in this world from those in the other world and the reception of religious and other types of instructions from those in the other world.

References

Canning, Ray R. 1965. "Mormon Return-from-the-Dead Stories, Fact or Folklore." *Utah Academy Proceedings* 42:29-37.

Crowther, Duane S. 1967. *Life Everlasting.* Salt Lake City, Utah: Bookcraft, Inc.

Hinckley, Bryant S. 1959. *The Faith of Our Pioneer Fathers.* Salt Lake City, Utah: Deseret Book Co.

Johnson, Peter E. 1920. "A Testimony." *Relief Society Magazine* 7 (8): 451-53.

Kübler-Ross, Elisabeth. 1969. *On Death and Dying.* New York, N.Y.: Macmillan.

Lundahl, Craig R. 1976. Personal interview.

Lundahl, Craig R. 1977. Personal interview.

Lundwall, Nels B. No date. *The Vision.* Salt Lake City, Utah: Bookcraft Pub. Co.

Moody, Raymond A. 1975. *Life After Life.* Covington, Ga.: Mockingbird Books.

Moody, Raymond A. 1977. *Reflections on Life After Life.* Covington, Ga.: Mockingbird Books.

Noyes, Russell, and Roy Kletti. 1976. "Depersonalization in the Face of Life-Threatening Danger: A Description." *Psychiatry* 39: 19-27.

O'Dea, Thomas F. 1957. *The Mormons.* Chicago, Ill.: University of Chicago Press.

Osis, Karlis, and Erlendur Haraldsson. 1977. "Deathbed Observations by Physicians and Nurses: A Cross-Cultural Survey." *Journal of the American Society for Psychical Research* 71 (3):237-59.

Sabom, M.B., and S. Kreutziger. 1977. "The Experience of Near Death." *Death Education* 1:195-203.

Snow, LeRoi C. 1919. "Raised from the Dead." *Improvement Era* 32 (12):973-74.

Stokes, Jeremiah. 1945. *Modern Miracles.* Salt Lake City, Utah: Bookcraft Inc.

Wilson, Lerona. 1915. "Work for the Dead as Taught by My Father and Others from the Spirit World." Typewritten copy.

Woodruff, Wilford. 1909. Leaves from My Journal. Salt Lake City, Utah: Deseret News.

11

Do Suicide Survivors Report
Near-Death Experiences?

Kenneth Ring and Stephen Franklin

SINCE THE PUBLICATION OF MOODY's (1975) best selling book, *Life After Life,* professional and lay audiences alike have become increasingly aware of and interested in the kind of experience which is said to occur when an individual lies close to death or has passed into a temporary state of "clinical" death. Moody's informal but influential research disclosed a common pattern of experiences (now usually labelled the near-death experience, or NDE) which includes, among other features, an overwhelming feeling of peace and well-being, a sense that one's consciousness has separated from one's body, a perception of moving through a dark tunnel or void, an encounter with (what Moody called) "a being of light," a panoramic life review, and awareness of the presence of deceased loved ones and a number of other transcendental elements. Moody's claim was that such NDEs usually had a profound impact on the experient, not the least of which was the removal of any fear of death.

Although Moody's methodology was not rigorous and his findings were not quantified, his contention that a transcendent experience, unfolding roughly in accord with the description given above, often occurs when an individual is close to death has now

Reprinted from *Omega* 12:191–208, by permission of the publisher and the authors. Copyright 1981–1982 by Baywood Publishing Company.

been repeatedly upheld in more systematic research with adequate documentation (Greyson and Stevenson, 1978, 1979; Noyes, 1979; Audette, 1979; Ring, 1980; Sabom) as well as in smaller-scale, more informal studies (Lundahl, 1979; Lee, 1978). The controversy over NDEs has continued to be concerned with their interpretation and significance (Rodin, 1980; Moody, 1980; Sabom, 1980; Schnaper, 1980; Stevenson, 1980; Ring, 1980; Blacher, 1980; Vicchio, 1979). Their occurrence, as such, as well as their after-effects, have now been amply attested to and are no longer in doubt.

In recent research on NDEs, attention has accordingly shifted away from simply providing more case history material to an interest in specifying the *determinants* of NDEs (Ring, 1980; Sabom). At issue here is the question of the *invariance* of this phenomenon across different modes of near-death onset. Within this context, there has been considerable speculation about what kind of near-death experiences, if any, might be associated with suicide attempts and what the after-effects of such experiences might be.

As Greyson's recent review makes clear, however, there are almost no research studies which bear on these issues, despite the voluminous literature on suicide itself. Aside from some extremely limited (though provocative) case history material (Rosen, 1975, 1976) and a few anecdotal accounts (Moody, 1975, 1977; Rawlings, 1978), there appears to have been no systematic research on these questions until Ring (1980) investigated them.

The purpose of this article is to present the combined results of two separate research projects dealing with the suicide question. We will supplement material from Ring's initial sample with the findings of a second study recently conducted jointly by the authors. Because the data-gathering procedure was identical for the two studies and the respondents comparable, it is both legitimate and expedient to consider our findings as constituting a single study of suicide-related near-death episodes. The therapeutic implications of our data will be discussed later in this report.

METHODS

Thirty-six persons who had been close to death as a result of a suicide attempt were interviewed using a structured interview schedule described elsewhere (Ring, 1980). The interview, which usually took place in the respondent's home, dealt with such matters as the circumstances of the suicide attempt, memories, if any, of the ensuing suicide-related experience, and after-effects stemming from the event. A number of questions were also asked of each respondent concerned with a comparison of certain beliefs and attitudes before and after the event. The entire interview took between one-half and one and one-half hours to complete and was tape recorded. Respondents were assured of confidentiality and anonymity.

The interviewees ranged in age from eighteen to fifty-eight with a mean age of about thirty-two. There were twenty-six females in the sample and ten males. Because of the difficulty in obtaining names of those who attempted suicide from the hospitals with which we were working (as part of larger investigation concerned with NDEs), we were obliged to advertise in local newspapers to obtain most of our cases (only nine—or one-quarter of our sample—were referred to us by our hospital sources). Our advertisements said that, as part of a University of Connecticut research project, we were interested to talk with anyone who had been close to death as a result of a suicide attempt. No mention was made of any special interest in a suicide-related experience as such, either in the advertisement or at the time of the interview. No monetary incentives were offered for participating in the study.

Because of the method of recruitment of most of our subjects, the matter of determining nearness to death deserves explicit comment. In our larger study of NDEs, it was usually possible to obtain the necessary information for hospital-referred near-death survivors in order to arrive at a reasonably secure judgment concerning an individual's closeness to death. This judgment was based on physicians' statements and medical records (where available) as well as on the testimony of the individual himself and (sometimes) members of his family. In the case of suicide survivors, however, such detailed information from other sources was often lacking and, as a result, we were obliged in many instances to rely primarily on the respondent's own assessment of his proximity to death.

Nevertheless, certain precautions were taken to minimize the risk that our sample would include individuals who had not actually been close to death. Ordinarily, the preliminary information we were able to gather about each potential respondent served a screening function. Individuals who appeared to have made merely a "suicidal gesture" and who did not lose consciousness were excluded from the study. In addition, anyone, however seriously intent on suicide he might have been, who indicated he did not feel that he had come close to death as a consequence of his suicide attempt was not interviewed. The outcome of this kind of preliminary screening was a sample of suicide survivors who, by and large, had lost consciousness—often for an extended period (up to four days)—and who felt they had either been close to death or, more rarely, experienced clinical death.

As a check on our selection criteria, each interviewee was rated by a panel of three judges on a five-point near-death scale, ranging from 0 (in no real danger of dying) to 4 (resuscitated; probably was clinically dead). The average of these ratings was 2.14 (2 = serious suicide attempt; probably would have died if condition persisted), and only two cases received average ratings of (slightly) less than 1 (serious suicide attempt, but not clear if individual would have died if condition persisted). Average inter-rater reliability for the first twenty-four cases was .65.

Thus, though the circumstances of our investigation precluded rigorous selection criteria or precise estimates of proximity to death, the bulk of our evidence (including that to be presented in the next section) is consistent with the contention that our sample of suicide survivors was composed preponderantly, if not exclusively, of persons who had come precariously close to death.

It must be stressed, however, that our respondents can in no way be considered a representative sample of suicide survivors. Nevertheless, since our interest was not to provide a parameter estimate of NDEs among such persons but only to determine whether they occur and conform to the classic NDE pattern, the sample of respondents we did obtain should be adequate to furnish us with preliminary answers to the issues of concern to us here.

Results

To determine objectively whether suicide survivors report NDEs, we evaluated each respondent's account using a measure of near-death experiences called the Weighted Core Experience Index. The derivation and rationale of this index has been explained elsewhere (Ring, 1980) and has been used by other investigators (Sabom, in press). Essentially, it provides a quantitative measure of the depth of a classic Moody-type NDE. Scores on the WCEI can range from 0 (indicating an absence of any NDE) to 29. Independent investigators (Ring, 1980; Sabom, in press) have found that a score of 6 or higher on this index is evidence that a Moody-type NDE occurred.

Using this cut-off point, we found that seventeen of our thirty-six respondents, or approximately 47 percent of our sample, reported such NDEs. This incidence among suicide attempters is not markedly different from that for other categories of near-death survivors. For example, in Ring's (1980) investigation, the percentage of near-death experiencers among illness and accident victims only was approximately 51 percent.

Table 1 shows the frequency of various elements commonly found in accounts of NDEs. All of these features have been found in previous research with other categories of near-death survivors, with only one possible minor exception to be noted later. Furthermore, although our sample of those attempting suicide is clearly too small to afford reliable comparisons, the percentage of cases reporting the various elements listed in Table 1 is generally in keeping with incidence figures for nonsuicide connected NDEs.

In short, our data suggest that suicide-related NDEs occur about as frequently as NDEs brought about in other ways and are composed of the same components. Simply put, then, there is nothing unique about NDEs triggered by suicide attempts.

Given the seeming invariance of NDEs, it is nevertheless still possible to ask: Does the way in which one attempts to take his life affect the likelihood of inducing an NDE? Unfortunately, our data do not permit a clear-cut answer to this question. Only a handful of our cases used methods other than drug overdose. All we can say is that no means of suicide-attempt precludes an NDE. We cannot yet say whether some means are more likely than others to induce one. Presumably the critical factor in most instances is coming close to death itself,[1] not the device used to arrive there.

Having focussed on the uniformities of NDEs so far, it is time to note some differences.

First of all, we found evidence of a possible sex difference in suicide-related NDEs. Eighty percent of the men who attempted suicide reported such experiences compared to approximately 35 percent of the women. This difference is significant ($\chi^2 = 4.29$,

---

[1] Nevertheless, it should be noted that Ring's (1980) previous work indicated that only a moderate relationship [r=.3] exists between the depth of an NDE (as measured by the WCEI) and estimates of closeness to death. In the suicide survivor sample described in this report, there was no difference in near-death estimates between those who reported an NDE and those who did not.

TABLE 1

Frequency and Percentage of NDE Elements in Suicide
Survivors Reporting an NDE (n = 17)

Element	n	percent
Feeling of peace and/or well-being	17	100
Having an out-of-body experience	7	41
Entering into a darkness or haze	9	53
Seeing a white or golden light	4	24
Encountering a "presence"	4	24
Experiencing a life review	4	24
Making a life decision or being told to return to life	6	35
Awareness of "another world"	4	24
Communicating with "spirits" of loved ones	4	24
Hearing beautiful music	2	12

$p<.05$). Furthermore, this is not the first time that sex differences in NDEs have been found (Ring, 1980). Nevertheless, it should be noted that although men exceeded women in the incidence of these NDEs, their WCEI scores were about the same and there were no important differences in the kind of NDE described.

Second, we found that NDEs associated with suicide attempts tended to fall into one of three relatively distinct patterns. Our findings here suggest that though these three patterns may separately represent stages of the NDE, they deserve to be differentiated from one another if one is to arrive at a clear understanding of the possible varieties of NDEs. In any case, by examining these patterns individually here, we will be able to gain a much keener qualitative "feel" for what someone attempting suicide may experience when he hovers on the edge of death.

Before delineating these three patterns, it is important to note, however, that they differ from one another chiefly in terms of their content, not their affect. The affective tone of all varieties of suicide-related NDEs tends to be extremely positive and most descriptions emphasize the peace, beauty and sense of perfection that usually accompany and pervade the experience of dying. A few brief quotes here will be sufficient to illustrate the strength of those feelings.

> I felt real good. I felt really peaceful, relaxed, a real mellow feeling. Everything was nice...nothing could happen to me any more.

> It was really beautiful and extremely peaceful.... The feelings—I've never had any feelings like that. It was just like knowing everything was right.

> It was a very cool, calm detached type of feeling, and at the same time it was a really free feeling. It was very pleasant and inspiring...it was beautiful.

> I have never forgotten the [pause] the peace and the love and the warmth, and there aren't any words to describe it. It just...was there, it was all consuming and I've never felt that since.

> A perfectly beautiful, beautiful feeling...to me, there's a definite feeling of sunlight and warmth associated with this peaceful feeling.... I felt warm, safe, happy, relaxed, just every wonderful adjective you could possibly use.

In this respect, the testimony of these suicide survivors is in no way different from that of others whose NDEs have been brought about by illness or accident (Ring, 1980). As Table 1 makes clear, all NDE respondents reported positive feelings, though not all to the same degree, and none described any negative ones in association with the experience itself.

NDE Type I: Out-of-Body Experience

The first variety of suicide-related NDEs is one which is characterized by a distinct sense that one's consciousness has separated from one's body. Typically the individual will state that he can see his physical body, as though he is a spectator to it, from a position above and to the side of his physical body, often "in the corner of the room." In most cases, one's vision is clear and although the room is sometimes perceived as illuminated very brightly, the whole situation is reported as distinctly real. The sense of hearing is also functional and is sometimes described as more acute than normal. Ordinarily, the individual relating such an out-of-body episode will not feel that he is "occupying" a second body; it is just that his "mind" is no longer "in" his body. To other observers, of course, the individual's body is either known or believed to be unconscious during this time and his eyes are closed.

Seven NDE respondents described this kind of experience and, significantly, none of them mentioned experiencing any other NDE features (to be discussed later) beyond the out-of-body episode itself. Excerpts from three illustrative cases will be presented next in order to convey something of the quality of Type I NDEs.

A twenty-one-year-old woman, after taking a large dose of anti-depressants, recounted her out-of-body experience as follows:

> The next thing I remember is being in intensive care.... I remember it from being in the corner of the room and I wasn't in my body.... I was definitely watching what was going on. I saw my body, and I saw nurses running in and out.... I definitely felt like I was out of my body. I wasn't aware of any kind of bodily sensations except warmth.

Later she tried to describe the quality of the light she perceived in the room while subjectively out of her body:

> It was a real bright mist. Mist is the closest but it wasn't wet. It just was really bright, but there was more than just light—there was substance to it, but there wasn't. Oh, God, it's hard to describe it! It was just all around me.... It was really beautiful.

In reflecting on the quality of her experience, she commented:

> It wasn't like a dream. I've had hallucinations with the drugs and it wasn't like that. It was a real, clear [pause] it was just as real, no—it was realer than being here right now. It was just very real, very clear.

A second instance comes from an interview with a twenty-eight year-old man. His suicide attempt followed a party where he had drunk alcohol laced with LSD. The following morning he slit his wrists, precipitating this experience:

> Somehow I was sitting in the corner of my room, and I can remember this clearly. [He describes various "objects in his room]... I was sitting in the far corner over there, next to the closet and there was a line, and my [physical] body was over here lying in a pool of blood, and I was sitting over there looking at myself saying, "What's that?" I didn't know where I was at first, and I can remember looking around and saying "this is nice" [and feeling] nice warmth from the sun.... I sensed the light that I assumed was sunlight and I felt the warmth... but there was no sun in that portion of the room.

Like the first respondent, he avers that his perception was marked by clarity and that his experience was unlike others which were drug-induced:

> I could see everything in the room clear as a bell, especially my body and the blood around it.... It wasn't a dream. [How about drugs?] No, it was very clear. It wasn't foggy or anything. It wasn't like smoking pot or being on acid or any of the drugs I've ever messed with. It was very clear.... In my view, it was not related to the drugs.

Almost as if to support this respondent's judgement is our last case in which an out-of-body experience was induced without drugs. Here a twenty-three-year-old woman had attempted suicide by jumping off a bridge onto a highway. After hitting the pavement, she recalled:

> ...being out of my body. I viewed my body all bloody. There were people all around me. I went back into my body and said, "Get me out of this blood." I remember someone saying to me, "We can't move you." [Later] I was out of my body viewing doctors, well, all these white [clothed] bodies, all around my body.... I must have been in a hospital room.

She described her out-of-body "position" as being in front of and above her physical body and also commented that the light in her hospital room seemed "very, very bright." She was uncertain whether the intensity of the illumination could be attributed to the lighting in the room itself.

NDE Type II: The Dark Void Experience

The second variety of suicide-related NDE involves primarily a sense of being pulled or feeling oneself drifting through a darkness (or, in one case, a grayness). The experience tends to be pleasant but lacking in specific elements. Respondents reporting this kind of NDE typically feel that they are "heading somewhere" but are "pulled back" before they arrive. Only two additional features are sometimes found here which are worth noting. The first is all but one of our four life-review cases fell into this category. The second feature is the perception of small "twinkly" or "shiny" lights as though off in the distance. My own provisional interpretation of the Type II NDE is that it represents a transitional experience lying between the out-of-body episodes characteristic of Type I NDEs and the more "other-worldly" experiences associated with Type III NDEs.

Five NDE respondents reported a Type II experience and, interestingly, none of these persons could recall having an out-of-body experience of the kind typical of Type I interviewees. Although most did report a feeling of a detachment from their physical bodies, no one said he could perceive it as though viewing it from outside himself. A few case history excerpts follow to illustrate the essentials of the Type II NDE.

A twenty-six-year-old woman, after a drug overdose, found that she:

> ...gradually sunk, floating, into this darkness.... I felt safe, protected and warm [in this darkness]. At one point I sort of remember a lot of air moving past me.... I just saw a lot of lights. Pinpricks. As though they were turned on in different places, like Christmas tree lights blinking on and off.

A more extended account of a Type II NDE comes from a twenty-five-year-old man who made several suicide attempts using a variety of drugs. The first time:

> ...all of a sudden I couldn't feel that I had a body. I felt like energy going into space. It was all total darkness, and I felt like a rush, like going into a pitch black place. It was just drawing me, drawing me, drawing me. Then, all of a sudden I felt a pull back, pull back, pull back.

Another time when he overdosed, he again:

> ...had that experience, only I experienced it twice.... It was the same thing, total darkness and I felt as if I were energy going off in one pattern toward darkness.... Everything just kept coming faster and faster, as if I was travelling off some place distant. I was heading toward a direction.... [Later] But then all of a sudden like little lights at a distance and I just kept going toward them. I experienced that the second time—lights in the distance. Lights or little sprinkles all over, shiny.... But then all of a sudden as I was going forward, it started bringing me back, back, back.

This man also reported a classic life review phenomenon (Ring, 1980; Noyes, 1977) and as to the reality of his experiences in general said simply, but with a touch of unintended irony, "it was so realistic, it was unbelievable."

The last example of a Type II experience is provided by the only person in this category to report drifting through a grayness rather than a blackness or darkness, as it is usually described. This is an instance of the possible minor variation, mentioned earlier, from other NDE accounts of this phenomenon inasmuch as it has occurred, to the best of our knowledge, only three times in all our NDE cases but each time in a suicide survivor. The reliability of this variation, in association with suicide cases, as well as its possible significance cannot be assessed without further research. In other respects this last case lends further support to our provisional interpretation that the Type II experience constitutes an interrupted journey.

A twenty-year-old man, after ingesting an assortment of drugs, found that he was at first aware only of floating through:

> ...grayness. Like I was in gray water or something. I couldn't really see anything. I couldn't see myself there either. It was just like my mind was there. And no body.

After experiencing a life review, he became aware of music which made him feel relaxed and gave him a feeling, a hope that he might be headed for someplace "better." After a while he became aware of a woman's voice:

> I just remember that it was a soothing voice...her voice kind of calling...my moving toward it...like that was the place to be....I kept trying to *get* where the voice was, but something was holding me back. I know I wanted to be there; I know once I was there everything would be fine. I was sure of this. No question about it. But there was still something holding me back from getting there.

Finally, the conflict was resolved: he was pulled back.

> The thing I remember most is a falling feeling. Like I was coming down really fast and then hit. And then I woke up with, like, a jolt.

NDE Type III: The "Other World" Experience

The last variety of suicide-related NDEs takes an individual beyond the (hypothesized) transitional stage we have just reviewed into "another world"—a realm of radiant light and preternatural beauty. Like Type II NDEs, these experiences do not include a consciously recalled out-of-body episode, but tend to begin with an experience of going through a dark tunnel or other opening. Unlike Type II NDEs, the "passage experience" seems to take one through an enclosure with a fairly definite configuration (in contrast to, say, "a darkness" characteristic of Type II NDEs). Golden or white light is usually seen at the end of this passageway and upon emerging from it, one (subjectively) finds himself in a world of surpassing beauty where the colors are notable for their vividness and intensity. Everything seems to be suffused in golden light. In addition to "natural scenery," there are "other beings" in this world. Some appear to be the "spirits" of deceased loved ones; others appear to be historical religious personages. Ordinarily, a telepathic conversation will take place between the individual and the being(s) he encounters. The upshot of this conversation invariably is that it is not the appropriate time for the individual to die and that he must "go back." In most cases, that injunction serves to terminate the Type III NDE.

Four suicide survivors gave Type III NDE accounts. Three cases involved drugs; the other, a fall. Because these individuals represent the most extended NDEs in our sample, with WCEI scores ranging from 13 to 25, an attempt will be made to summarize, using interview excerpts, the essentials of each person's experience. It needs to be borne in mind, however, that because these are very complex episodes, this sort of summary is perhaps least satisfactory for Type III NDEs. Indeed, each account contains such an abundance of relevant content and important nuance that only the full transcript would do full justice to it.

A forty-four-year-old woman reported that her experience began with:

> ...a roar and a tunnel and spinning and it suddenly was like lightning hit and my [deceased] uncle was there and I remember embracing him and he smiled.

After describing her feelings of peace, love and warmth (quoted earlier), she next related an encounter with "three beings" who were "very, very white and very glowing" with bodies "enshrouded in this moving gold." One of them told her, "You must go back." At this point, she said:

> I started to scream because I was moving backwards or wherever I was being pulled away.... Moving away was like a suction, picking up speed, like being in a vacuum tube, you know, but you're there and there's not much you can do about it. I was just furious, then, yes. I didn't want to come back.

Later, she amplified on certain features of her experience. About her tunnel experience, she said:

> There was a pinhole light at first and the roar picked up and I remember just going right through the light, and I was there, just as easy as that. [The light] was blinding... it's like being in a subway and coming out of a tunnel. The strange thing is that once I got into it I didn't have to squint. I was part of it.

On the colors:

> Colors are very totally flat here, but they were very vivid and alive and real there. They had almost like an electrical charge. Everything. The golds and the blues, my uncle himself was more vibrant and he was a lot younger.

Finally, on the reality of the experience itself:

> ...it was very real; I couldn't deny that.

The second case is that of a thirty-two-year-old man who had taken an overdose of tranquillizers. He recalled:

> I remember going through this white grayish sandish haze and it opened up and everything was a desert—like grayish sand. And in the middle of this was a black stick... that was the only thing there. So I started walking up to this—and it felt pretty good—to this object and I got to it and what it was—I would say it was Jesus Christ; I mean it looked like Him. He was dressed in a robe that was a robin's egg blue, and a long flowing robe that wrapped around Him and He had this staff that was a bright gold. It must have been ten feet high. I was looking at Him. We were having a conversation. If I could ever put my mind into the space I was in there and know what we were talking about, I'm sure I would really have a lot of satisfactory feelings about a lot of questions that I've been wondering about....[As to the conversation] I can't remember it, but I was really comfortable talking and whatever it was, I agreed with it. There wasn't any unpleasant feelings during the whole experience.

Later he commented:

> Vision was clear, everything that was there stood out.... The colors had a brilliance, this whole person had a brilliance or an aura about Him.... It was probably the happiest I've ever been.

And as for skeptics:

> Going through an experience like that, afterwards it just puts a belief into you that no matter what anybody says or whoever tries to disqualify these, it will never hold up with me because I believe I have seen something of where I'm eventually going....

The next case is based on the report of a twenty-eight-year-old man who, while in jail, dove head first from an eight-foot platform onto a cement floor. Immediately, he said:

[I] heard all this ringing, this loud, loud ringing and then a black hole and all these luminous things around and beautiful music, the most beautiful music I had ever heard.... The ringing came from a low to a peak which faded into choral music, which was all around me. It was the most beautiful experience I think I've ever had, just totally encompassed in sound, the most beautiful voices I'd ever heard.

He then noticed an enclosure from which emanated light. He was drawn to it, feeling that there was someone there whom he knew. He saw "beings" there:

I saw white silk type gowns, just sort of a flowing thing, no real substance to them, but there was substance to them. It was sort of an ether state, very, very, light, delicate and sturdy. They were singing.... I just sort of looked around for a while and then either a voice or a being [he thinks it might have been his deceased grandfather] said, "Take to your body." I said, "I don't want to." He said, "You've got to, you've got other things to do," then I went back into my body, maybe through my solar plexus area. Everything was just so bright, white gold, luminous beings—and then I was sucked back into my body.

The last case here is that of a twenty-eight-year-old woman who, as a teenager, swallowed an entire bottle of aspirin tablets. Following a panoramic life review, she, too, remembers:

...going down into this big black tunnel, just twirling and twirling... and after a while my ears were starting to ring....The tunnel was pretty dark, pretty black, but you could sense, like, stars....[Then] it was hard to look at because it was extremely bright, you know, after being in a dark area and then all of a sudden you're looking into this great white light. And it was warm. I know because I was cold as I was going through the tunnel and then when I hit the other side and as I approached this light, you could feel the difference in temperature—extremely warm.

She then became aware of a beautiful vista before her which, somehow, she could not enter but only perceive. It consisted of:

...fields and flowers, mountains—things like that. Beautiful, all beautiful. [Asked about the colors, she said] Oh yeah, blues, whites, daisies, all kinds of flowers, really beautiful.

Afterwards, however, as with some of the respondents we have already quoted:

> It's all of a sudden being picked up, and I had no choice, all of a sudden I'm flying [back] through this tunnel, and I was falling... and falling... and the speed picked up—it was a tremendous force.

Unlike our other respondents, though, her NDE experience does not end with her return. Before she regained consciousness, she again perceived a white light:

> I could feel this white light around my head and then it started to move over to here where I could see it on the side, and it started talking to me. I was flabbergasted... it was my great grandmother who had died maybe a year, two years [before].

She reported that her great-grandmother exhorted her to see that "things were not that bad" and that she, the great grandmother, could be called upon in times of trouble. When the respondent protested and said she wanted to return to where she had been before, she was told that she couldn't, that it wasn't her time. After that, the experience faded out and she awoke to ordinary consciousness feeling extremely sick.

All but one of our cases fit into the trichotomous classification system we have used as a framework to delineate the major varieties of suicide-related NDEs. The remaining case involved an encounter with what the respondent took to be God, but it did not otherwise conform to the features associated with Type III NDEs.

For purposes of comparison of suicide-related NDEs with naturally occurring NDEs, it is necessary to refer to one last set of data available from our sample of suicide survivors. These are the data on aftereffects. Since this study is primarily concerned with the phenomenology of suicide attempts, however, and since the data on aftereffects are, as will be imagined, rich and complex in their own right, only a brief summary of them will be offered here—and that chiefly with the aim of cross-NDE comparisons in mind. We shall consider these aftereffects at length in a subsequent report.

Ring's (1980) previous work revealed a general increase in religiousness following an NDE compared to near-death survivors who could recall no experience. Among suicide survivors, we found a similar trend, but it was not statistically significant. Like those undergoing NDEs in general, however, suicide survivors reporting an NDE show a significantly greater increase in belief in life after death compared to nonexperiencers (t = 2.53, p<.02). Finally, we have some inconclusive but highly suggestive data to report on the reduction of the fear of death. In general, it has been found (Ring 1980; Sabom 1982) that those undergoing an NDE show a sharp decline in fear of death following their experience whereas nonexperiencers tend to remain the same. In our study, we were able to inquire into this matter using a quantitative index of change only for our last thirteen respondents, ten NDEers and three non-experiencers. Everyone undergoing an NDE showed a decline in fear of death (usually stating that they now feared death not at all) except for one who, both before and afterward, said she was unafraid of death. However, two nonexperiencers also evinced similar declines; but one nonexperiencer showed a substantial increase in fear following her suicide attempt. It remains to be seen, then, how much just surviving a suicide attempt per se reduces fear of death and how much of an effect, if any, is added by having an NDE during one's suicide episode. Of course, it may well be that those who attempt suicide have less fear of death to begin with than those who never attempt suicide. If so, we might have reason not to expect comparable effects here, compared to other categories of near-death survivors. In any event, more research is needed to clarify this matter.

DISCUSSION

The findings from the present investigation strongly support the invariance hypothesis concerning NDEs. That is, however NDEs are brought about, the experience itself is much the same. As we have seen, the same elements that comprise NDEs triggered by illness and accident were reported by persons surviving a suicide attempt. Furthermore, the proportion of suicide survivors who claimed to undergo an NDE was roughly the same as that of other categories of near-death survivors, although, to be sure, our sample may not be representative of those who come close to death as a result of a suicide attempt.

Although implicit in the foregoing comments, it should probably be emphasized here that not one suicide survivor reported an experience that was predominantly unpleasant. No one felt that he either was in or was bound for hell. Quite the contrary: suicide-related NDEs were usually quite pleasant and beautiful, often exceedingly so, as we have indicated. Only when an individual found himself returning—often against his will—to physical life did his affective response change to the negative. Moreover, during the NDE itself no one felt himself to be judged, much less condemned, by any force outside himself for his suicidal action.

Needless to say, near-death research can never settle the question of whether there is a hell any more than its findings can prove the existence of any sort of afterlife.

It is clear that our data offer no support to the claims of such researchers as Rawlings (1978) that suicide-induced NDEs will be unpleasant. We are not of course asserting that negative NDEs cannot occur—only that we found none. Actually, our findings are much more consistent with those of Rosen (1975, 1976) who found abundant evidence for transcendental experiences of a highly positive kind.

The conceptualization of NDEs, however, is a matter to which our data appear to be highly relevant. It will be recalled that among our suicide survivors we found evidence for three discrete patterns of NDEs. All NDE patterns were associated with highly positive effect but differed significantly in content.

There appear to be two principal ways in which these NDEs may be understood. One possibility is simply to take them at face value. Rather than assuming that the NDE is a uniform experience, as Moody's (1975) work originally suggested, it may be that NDEs actually unfold according to one of several distinct progressions. A second possibility is based on Ring's (1980) five stage sequential model of NDEs. This model states that NDEs tend to progress from the out-of-body stage through the dark void or tunnel to the light and entrance into "another world." Thus, this model posits a fundamental continuity and implies that the various NDE patterns delineated here are merely discrete stages of an underlying progression. The present data raise two difficulties for the Ring model, however, which need to be noted here. They are: (1) why should Type II and III respondents never report a clear out-of-body experience? and (2) why should Type I respondents never progress beyond the out-of-body experience? Either these effects (assuming they are replicated) are unique to suicide attempts in which case the model has limited validity or the model has no validity whatever. Only further research, with both suicide survivors and other varieties of near-death survivors, can resolve the issue of how we can best conceptualize the NDE.

Several other questions about suicide-related NDEs raised but not settled by the present investigation also need to be addressed in future research. We shall simply enumerate them, commenting briefly where necessary.

1. Does the mode of suicide attempt affect the likelihood, depth or content of the NDE? Although our work demonstrated that suicide-related NDEs can occur without drugs, the role of drugs in this connection needs to be further examined. Especially relevant here is the research of Osis and Haraldsson (1977) which suggests that certain aspects of NDEs are inhibited rather than facilitated by drugs.
2. Are there sex differences in the incidence of suicide-related NDEs?
3. Is there evidence that a "gray mist" or "gray area" as part of the transition experience is unique to suicide survivors?
4. What are the effects of suicide episodes, with and without accompanying NDEs, on suicide survivors' attitude toward and fear of death? Do people who attempt suicide fear death less than others to begin with?

In the remainder of this section, we shall be concerned with a discussion of the therapeutic implications of our research findings, especially in the light of some of our respondents' views of the suicidal act following their own suicide-related NDE.

The fear has been expressed (Schneidman, 1971) that ideas which tend to romanticize death by implying some sort of glorified existence following death may actually increase the incidence of suicide attempts. Clearly the findings of near-death research in general and studies such as ours in particular are vulnerable to this criticism. Although, as we have said, near-death research can obviously never prove there is a life after death, much less that that life is always an improvement over earthly life, it is obvious that near-death research does tend to convey a very positive idea of a possible afterlife. People whose desire to quit this life is strong and whose suicidal longing exceeds their scientific judgment might certainly find their suicidal temptations increased after reading such NDE accounts as those provided by this paper.

But only if they stop reading here!

The fact is that, however plausible this line of reasoning may be, it appears to be wrong. The following comments will show why.

According to Greyson's very valuable consideration of this issue, the available evidence, though admittedly scanty, suggests that there is actually a decrease in suicidal intent following a suicide-induced NDE. In fact, he states that there is in the literature he has reviewed not a single case thus far reported of suicidal intent persisting or increasing following an NDE. While he rightly urges caution in interpreting these findings and calls for more research on the question, the implication of his argument is that it is chiefly those suicide attempters who do not undergo an NDE who are likely to try again—not those who report an NDE.

Our findings strongly support Greyson's thesis. Although we can only summarize our data here (pending a full report on a subsequent publication), we can say that the common testimony among those we interviewed who had an NDE was that, in most cases, suicide had ceased to be an option. The modal response was that though they did indeed value—even treasure—their NDE, they would not recommend to anyone else that he take this means to try to achieve one nor were they tempted to try for one again in this way. More than this, several of our respondents stated that they would be willing to counsel others against suicide despite (or, perhaps one should say, because of) having had a beautiful suicide-related NDE themselves. (We shall consider some possible reasons for this counter-intuitive effect shortly.)

Thus, if suicidal individuals pay heed to the real authorities—those who have been there—the result of publicizing these suicide-related NDEs should actually serve to deter rather than to promote suicide attempts. If so, then merely the dissemination of this material, along with suicide attempters' own views, can in itself be regarded as a therapeutic measure.

Not only do suicide survivors who report an NDE tend to discourage suicide but so also do others who have undergone an NDE brought about in other ways. Ring (1980) has provided some relevant material here and Greyson and Stevenson (1978) have also shown that negative attitude changes toward suicide are correlated with feelings of peacefulness or contentment during an NDE.

In short, the recollective testimony of suicide survivors and other near-death survivors alike is that the NDE, rightly interpreted, promotes the cause of life, not death, and especially not death via a suicide attempt.

Intuitively, this outcome seems paradoxical and certainly confounds the expectations of many who might otherwise feel that near-death research findings could provoke a rash of suicides. We would like to suggest, however, that a deeper examination rather than a facile dismissal of the NDE will both eliminate the sense of paradox about the effects of such experiences and provide the basis for a more balanced view.

How, then, to interpret the NDE? Although Ring (in press) has recently proposed a theory for understanding the transformative effects of NDEs in general, we shall phrase our interpretation here in terms of the notions of ego-death and transcendence.

Grof and Halifax (1977) have proposed that a key transformative event in mystical states of consciousness, whether induced or spontaneous, is what they term an ego-death. Essentially, this is a shattering emotional experience in which an individual "dies to himself" in such a way that ordinary ego functioning is disrupted or absent. In this state the individual typically becomes aware of a higher transcendent order. Grof and Halifax state that such experiences are always followed by feelings of rebirth and that individuals plunged into an ego-death experience "usually become open to the possibility that consciousness might be independent of the physical body and continue beyond the moment of clinical death" (p. 52).

We suggest that something analogous happens in NDEs: functionally, they, too, bring about an ego-death and instill a sense that one's consciousness will survive death.

In the case of suicidal individuals, Grof and Halifax advance the hypothesis that what they are really seeking is transcendence, not death as such. And the implication of their argument is that when a transcendent experience is achieved, not only are suicidal tendencies diminished but positive appreciation of life is enhanced. Certainly that seems to have been the case in Rosen's (1975, 1976) study of those few individuals who survived suicidal leaps from the Golden Gate and Oakland-San Francisco Bay Bridge. In his work, he clearly demonstrates the transcendent nature of these suicidal experiences and invokes the concept of "egocide" to understand them. Greyson also is partial to this notion of egocide. So are we. And we believe that suicide-related NDEs tend to engender this condition with all of its life-enhancing potentials.

The transformations that come about in the lives of near-death survivors tend to be dramatic and profound (Ring, 1980) and this includes those who attempt suicide who experience an NDE. Again, there seems to be an invariance here: however the NDE is brought about it tends to have much the same effect. When one has a subjectively undeniable view of the beauty of the cosmos and comes to understand that one is indissolubly a part of it, the means by which that insight is achieved becomes irrelevant. It only remains to return to physical life and to try to live in accordance with the knowledge one has gleaned while on the threshold of death.

Whatever the ontological validity of this view of human existence, it is the understanding that most suicide survivors, who have had NDEs, seem to have of their experience. It makes it clear why their common interpretation and advice can only serve to promote life, not subvert it.

Clinical psychologists like McDonagh (1979) have already been able to make effective use of the knowledge of NDEs to discourage suicide attempts. It is to be hoped that the direct testimony of suicide survivors themselves can be used even more successfully toward this end.

References

Audette, J. 1979. "Denver Cardiologist Discloses Findings After 18 Years of Near-Death Research." *Anabiosis* 1:1-2.

Blacher, R.S. 1980. "To Sleep, Perchance to Dream...." *JAMA* 242:2291.

Greyson, B., and I. Stevenson. 1978. "Near-Death Experiences: Characteristic Features." Paper presented at the Parapsychology Association Conference, August, St. Louis, Mo. Submitted to the *American Journal of Psychiatry.*

Greyson, B. "Near-Death Experiences and Attempted Suicide." Submitted to the *American Journal of Psychiatry.*

Grof, S. and J. Halifax. 1977. *The Human Encounter with Death.* New York: Dutton.

Lee, A. 1978. "The Lazarus Syndrome: Caring for Patients Who've 'Returned from the Dead.'" *RN,* June 1978, pp. 53-64.

Lundahl, C. 1979. "The Near-Death Experiences of Mormons." Paper presented at the American Psychological Association convention, September, New York, N.Y.

McDonagh, J. 1979. "Bibliotherapy with Suicidal Patients." Paper presented at the American Psychological Association convention, September, New York, N.Y.

Moody, R.A., Jr., 1980. "Commentary on 'The Reality of Death Experiences: A Personal Perspective' by Ernst Rodin." *J. Nerv. Ment. Dis.* 168:264–65.

_____. 1975. *Life After Life.* Atlanta: Mockingbird Books.

_____. 1977. *Reflections on Life After Life.* Atlanta: Mockingbird Books.

Noyes, R., Jr. 1977. "Panoramic Memory: A Response to the Threat of Death." *Omega* 8:181-94.

_____. 1979. "Near-Death Experiences: Their Interpretation and Significance." In R. Kastenbaum (Ed.), *Between Life and Death.* N.Y.: Springer.

Osis, K., and E. Haraldsson. 1977. *At the Hour of Death.* New York: Avon.

Rawlings, M. 1978. *Beyond Death's Door.* New York: Thomas Nelson.

Ring, K. 1980. "Comments on 'The Reailty of Death Experiences: A Personal Perspective' by Ernst A. Rodin." *J. Nerv. Ment. Dis.* 168:273-74.

_____. 1980. *Life at Death: A Scientific Investigation of the Near-Death Experience.* New York: Coward, McCann and Geoghegan.

_____. In press. "Near-Death Experiences: From Transcendence to Transformation." *J. Acad. Rel. Psychical Res.*

Rodin, E.A. 1980. "The Reality of Death Experiences: A Personal Perspective." *J. Nerv. Ment. Dis.* 168:259-63.

_____. 1980. "Commentary on 'The Reality of Death Experiences: A Personal Perspective' by Ernst Rodin." *J. Nerv. Ment. Dis.* 168:264-65.

Rosen, D.H. 1975. "Suicide Survivors." *West. J. Med.* 122:289-94.

_____. 1976. "Suicide Survivors: Psychotherapeutic Implications of Egocide." *Suicide and Life-Threatening Behavior* 6:209-15.

Sabom, M.B. 1980. "Commentary on 'The Reality of Death Experiences' by Ernst Rodin." *J. Nerv. Ment. Dis.* 168:266-67.

_____. 1982. *Recollections of Death.* New York: Harper and Row.

Schnaper, N. 1980. "Comments Germane to the Paper Entitled 'The Reality of Death Experiences' by Ernst Rodin." *J. Nerv. Ment. Dis.* 168:268-70.

Schneidman, E.S. 1971. "On the Deromanticization of Death." *Amer. J. Psychother.* 25:4-17.

Stevenson, I. 1980. "Comments on 'The Reality of Death Experiences: A Personal Perspective.'" *J. Nerv. Ment. Dis.* 168:271-72.

Stevenson, I., and B. Greyson. 1979. "Near-Death Experiences." *JAMA* 242:265-67.

Vicchio. S.J. 1979. "Against Raising Hope of Raising the Dead: Contra Moody and Kübler-Ross." *Essence* 3:51-67.

PART FOUR

Explanations for
Near-Death Experiences

12

Toward an Explanation of Near-Death Phenomena

Michael Grosso

THE HUMAN CONCEPT OF DEATH HAS undergone radical changes with the gradual waning and repression of archaic modes of thought. Early man lived in a world under the sway of the magical omnipotence of thought; moreover, the modern, post-Renaissance man's narrow and mechanized sense of self was unknown to the first people in the childhood of the human race. Orthodox science's view of death is not the view of primitives or of people of the great religious traditions. To the typical scientist, consciousness is the by-product of brain events and perishes with the body. Nevertheless, let us bracket this dogma for a moment and ask: Is death really the extinction of human personality or does it permit some continuity of consciousness? One purpose of what follows is to insist that this deserves to remain an open question, for the evidence suggesting survival is neither so compelling nor the dogmas which deny it so commanding that one can judge on the issue with much confidence.

A complex set of phenomena associated with near-death states seems at first glance to clash with the scientifically orthodox view of death as extinction. Scientists investigating these phenomena refer to them collectively as near-death experiences (NDEs). I want, first, to call the reader's attention to certain features of these experiences which demand explanation; we will then look at some of the explanations that have already been proposed and try to evaluate them impartially. At the very least, classic NDEs suggest some rather bizarre capabilities of the human mind; on that score alone they deserve to be studied by students of human behavior. On the other hand, they may turn out to be the foothills of a new frontier of knowledge.

TYPES OF NEAR-DEATH EXPERIENCE

There are two types of NDE. The first consists of deathbed visions. Here the subject typically is ill, usually bedridden, and suddenly at the hour of death experiences a vision. He often "sees" the apparition of a deceased relative or friend. The experience may be accompanied by a remarkable elevation of mood. The dying person is frequently in a state of clear, wakeful consciousness, and the apparition seems to inhabit, or temporarily manifest in, the space near the patient. Early collections of these cases were compiled and studied by Bozzano (1906, 1923), Hyslop (1908), and Barrett (1926). More recently, Osis (1961) took up the question of deathbed visions, and Osis and Haraldsson (1977a,b) pursued the problem using a cross-cultural approach.

In the second type of NDE a person, not necessarily ill, is suddenly brought into a state on the verge of physical death. This might arise from cardiac arrest, near drowning, mountain-climbing falls, suicide attempts, auto accidents, or other life-threatening incidents. Moody (1975) has constructed a model of this type of near-death experience. The main common elements in the experience are ineffability, feelings of peace and quiet, entering a dark tunnel, being out of the body, meeting with others, encountering a being of light, reaching a border or limit, and undergoing changes in outlook and attitude. The subsequent work of Ring (1980) largely supports the informal studies of Moody (1975, 1977). Ring describes five stages of a "prototypical" core experience: euphoric affect, an out-of-body state, entering darkness, seeing an unearthly world of light, and entering into that world of light. These stages seem like parts of an ordered and developing sequence in which subjects reach the final stages with decreasing frequency. At any one of these stages there might occur what Ring calls a "decisional process." The person "decides" to return to life. However, many cases involve anger or regret over being brought back to life; the process appears to be quite automatic. As Ring points out, we seem to be observing a prototypical or suprapersonal mechanism which manifests in a fragmentary way through a spectrum of personalities.

In addition to the five stages and the decisional process, Ring's cases include other features of classic near-death experiences such as meeting with others, panoramic memory, and so forth. On the whole, features of the two types of NDE, deathbed visions and close-call or resuscitation cases, are not inconsistent.

In a large number of the resuscitation cases the patient temporarily ceases to display any vital signs. But can we say that such patients were "really" dead? The problem is that during the period of the patient's "death," the organism was still capable of being restored to vital functioning. But we cannot say this of the body of someone who has died "permanently"; so in this sense the resuscitated patient was clearly not dead. On the other hand, the patient, having temporarily lost all vital functioning, would in the great majority of cases soon have joined the ranks of the permanently and irrevocably dead had it not been for the intervention of on-the-scene medical workers. In this sense, one is tempted to say that the resuscitated patient really was dead.

The fact that resuscitated patients would, without medical intervention, have died seems rather difficult to reconcile with their having any experience whatsoever. Suppose one dies in the sense that, apart from resuscitation procedures, one would remain irreversibly dead. Once that process has begun, what biological function can we ascribe to having any experiences—no less the extraordinary near-death experiences? As long as the organism is functioning vitally, however imminent death may be, it seems less surprising that the brain might throw off some adaptive phenomena —phantasms, memories, deliria. But once the first irreversible step is taken and the brain is rapidly depleting its last store of oxygen and glucose, it seems like an overstated and perfunctory gesture to go on producing such elaborate and useless epiphenomena.

THREE CLASSES OF PUZZLING EFFECTS

Three components of NDEs have to be explained: (1) the consistency and universality which they generally display, (2) their paranormal (psi) aspects, and (3) their power to modify attitudes and behavior.

The Consistency and Universality of NDEs

For the phenomenologist or student of the natural history of the mind, the NDE appears as a distinctive finding; a coherent, spontaneous psychic mechanism. The firsthand accounts arise from the most diverse sources—religious believers and atheists, the educated and the ignorant; from old and young, saint and sinner, man and woman. In case after case the same message, though coded differently and in accents and styles that vary, seems to emanate from a universal stratum of consciousness. What appears is a cross-cultural pattern of phenomena that is filtered down and personalized by the individual's inherited cultural constructs. For example, as Osis and Haraldsson (1977a,b) and Ring (1980) have found, religious beliefs influence the interpretation, not the content of the experience. Lundahl (elsewhere in this book) has studied near-death experiences of Mormons, some of which date back a hundred years, and found the core phenomena I have described above. Crookall (1965) has collected large numbers of cases, rich in descriptive detail, which again reinforce the reality of the core phenomena. For further historical studies supporting the consistency and universality of the core phenomena, see Audette's article in this book and Rogo (1979).

Moreover, there seem to be aspects of the NDE which are manifested in contexts which are not directly related to pathology or life-threatening situations: for instance, in dreams (Russell, 1965), mystical experiences (Noyes, 1971), esoteric death-training techniques (Evans-Wentz, 1957), psychedelic therapy with terminal patients (Grof and Halifax, 1977), and mystery cults of antiquity (Grosso, 1979). Needless to say, more work needs to be done to substantiate the claim of universality; nevertheless, the widespread pattern of the phenomena under examination calls for an explanation.

The Paranormal Aspects of NDEs

The second component that needs explanation is the paranormal material sometimes reported in NDEs. Most of this material is anecdotal, but the cumulative effect strongly suggests that there is some substance to the psi-dimension of these experiences. Further support comes from the evidence that altered states of consciousness are psi-conducive (see, for example, Honorton, 1977). This point is important because near-death situations generate altered states of consciousness.

The psi-components lend weight to the meaningful and consistent features of NDEs in two ways. First, they indicate that NDEs express more than just wish-fulfillment or self-serving fantasy. To the extent that such experiences contain elements of genuine psi, they are oriented toward objective reality. Secondly, psi in general suggests the existence of an alternate, nonsensory reality—a reality which could be construed in terms relevant to post-mortem states. This second point is of course controversial. But the facts about psi persist in being inexplicable in terms of physical theory (Beloff, 1980); they seem to imply the existence of an autonomous psychological order of reality. This should be kept in mind in trying to understand the wider implications of near-death phenomena.

Of course, there is nothing to prevent us from assuming that any psi components found in NDEs result from delusive expectations and irrational desires. This psi-dependent Freudian interpretation will have to be considered later. For now let us briefly examine some of the types of ostensible near-death-related psi effects, for it is these effects which sharpen the challenge of near-death phenomena.

Psi Effects Related to Deathbed Visions. In so-called "Peak in Darien" cases, the dying person sees the apparition of a person not known by the former to be deceased. If this is what it appears to be, we could describe it as a kind of transworld ESP. There are a few reports (Barrett, 1926; Bozzano, 1906) of cases in which nobody present was aware that the person whose apparition was seen was in fact dead, thus ruling out telepathy from people at the dying person's bedside. Cases of this type are rare, but this is not surprising in view of the peculiar combination of factors necessary to produce them. Unfortunately, most of the Peak in Darien cases derive from the older literature, though Lundahl in this book and Ring (1980, p. 208) offer some current illustrations. The impersonal nature of dying in modern hospitals may account for the dearth of recent examples.

Psi Effects Related to Resuscitation Cases. In resuscitation cases, or other types of near-death encounters, the dominant psi component comes in the form of ostensibly genuine out-of-body experiences (OBEs). Not all OBEs, of course, contain psi components. Yet there seems to be an almost typical report of a classic out-of-body situation in which a person near death finds himself located outside his body and able to observe in detail events occurring in neighboring regions of space. Cases such as this, assuming they can be corroborated, strongly suggest paranormal OB perception, though in any single instance ad hoc normal explanations could be invoked. In order to substantiate such claims of ND-related paranormal OB perception, it will be necessary in the future to obtain the cooperation of medical professionals. Obviously this will not be an easy task, given the stringent duties of physicians and nurses on the job. Yet much could be learned if psi investigation could be routinely incorporated into certain medical settings where one might suppose a gold mine of useful data awaits exploration.

As far as I know, Michael Sabom, a cardiologist working at the Emory University School of Medicine, Atlanta, is the first physician actively concerned with investigating the paranormal elements of NDEs. As an example[1] of an OBE with a possible psi component, Sabom has described a case in which a patient anesthetized for open-heart surgery, after a period of black-out—called "entering the darkness" by Ring and "the tunnel" by Moody and Crookall—suddenly became aware of his body being operated upon. The patient's face was covered by a sheet, yet he claims to have observed the operation from a point out of and above his body, as if he were another person, an unconcerned observer. The patient described how the "shining metal" of the knife cut through his chest, the syringes inserted on each side of his heart, and the injection into it. He watched a physician cut off bits of his heart, poke around some veins and arteries, and then discuss with other physicians where the next bypass was to be made. He observed a doctor wearing blood-stained white shoes, another with a bloodclot in the fingernail of his right hand.

Two observations particularly struck Sabom from his perspective as a cardiologist. The patient expressed surprise at the large size and actual location of his heart; he compared its shape to the continent of Africa. According to Sabom, this is an apt comparison. The patient also said that part of his heart had a lighter color than the normal myocardial tissue; according to Sabom, discoloration would have marked the site of the patient's previous heart attack.

Such apparently genuine OBEs need to be explained; they lend some weight to the unverifiable visionary claims of near-death or dying percipients. For, if one aspect of the NDE is verifiable while at the same time providing testimony for an extraphysical factor, then it seems less implausible to ascribe ultimately verifiable reality to the rest of the experience.

There are also reports of OBEs in deathbed vision cases. But here the apparent separation process may be more gradual. Osis and

Haraldsson (1977b, p. 129) write: "While still functioning normally, the patient's consciousness might be gradually disengaging itself from the ailing body." And in Barrett's (1926) early study, witnesses are cited who have "seen" dying persons' "doubles" splitting off and disappearing at the moment of death. These observations might explain why terminal patients often experience a lessening of pain and discomfort shortly before they die.

The dying patient may only be approaching the state that the resuscitated patient has already entered; yet there still seem to be gradations of entering more deeply into the NDE, as the work of Ring (1980) shows. Obviously, more has to be done on this "stage of entry" idea. One approach might be to obtain information on the dreams and mentations of people just prior to their sudden death or onset of fatal illness. For example, I have recorded several cases of individuals who, a day or so before a sudden fatal illness, unaccountably started to talk about their deceased relatives, had slips of the tongue suggesting subconscious preoccupation with them, spontaneously put their affairs in order, settled accounts, etc., as if in preparation for death.

Psychokinetic phenomena have also been reported in the context of death and dying. Bozzano (1948) made a study of psychokinetic (PK) events in conjunction with the time of death. Osis and Haraldsson (1977b, p. 42) referred to a few tantalizing incidents— for example, the stopping of clocks belonging to two of Thomas Alva Edison's associates and also of his own clock within moments of his death. And L.E. Rhine (1970, pp. 330-34) cites several interesting cases of PK effects associated with the dying and the dead, taken from her collection of spontaneous cases on file at the Institute for Parapsychology.

Finally, as further evidence bearing on the psi-conducive nature of death and dying, there is the S.P.R. Census of Hallucinations (Sidgwick and Committee 1894, p. 393), which showed that veridical apparitions "which coincide in time with the death of the person seen"—i.e., the "agent"—are more numerous than apparitions in any other category.

Changes in Outlook and Behavior

We observe in both types of NDEs a modification of outlook, affective states, values, and goals. This constitutes the third component of these experiences that calls for explanation. In the deathbed cases such effects are obviously of short duration because the patient dies shortly after the experience. Nevertheless, Osis and Haraldsson (1977a, 1977b) found cases of near-death rise of mood that could not be explained by medical factors. Sabom (1980) did follow-up studies six months after his patients' experiences and found that the modification effects persisted. Generally, it would appear that the near-death syndrome produces beneficial effects— in some respects resembling religious conversion. Chief among these effects is the reduction or elimination of the fear of death and alterations in outlook concerning the meaning of life and the nature of reality. The true benefits of these transformative experiences may, however, be blocked because of the confusion they elicit; patients are often unable to share their experiences and even fear for their sanity. Hopefully, with a better understanding of these phenomena the medical establishment will learn to enhance their utility. In sum, such near-death enhancement effects need to be explained because their adaptive potential seems incongruous with thinking of them as illusory or pathological.

EXPLAINING NEAR-DEATH EXPERIENCES

For an explanation of the NDE to work, it must address itself to all three components of the phenomenon: its universality and consistency; its paranormal dimension; and its transformative effects, which are usually of a positive nature. It is the unique combination of these components which makes it a challenging matter to explain the NDE. Obviously, the mere fact that a phenomenon is universal and consistent in itself need not impress us; drunkards of all cultures and personality types, for example, consistently have the same sort of experiences—say, delirium tremens. Consistency and universality here is no bar to seeing the drunkard's experience as delusory. But it is a different matter with near-death experiences, for we do not expect delusory experiences to produce momentous changes in personality or to involve extensions of normal human capabilities.

Methods of Gathering Data

Scientific research in NDE is still in its infancy. Most of the work so far has consisted of collecting reports unsystematically from pre-selected sources. Little or no medical and psychological data were included in the early collections of cases. The first systematic approach was that of Osis (1961), who used modern sampling techniques and computer analyses to sort out the patterns in his data. The recent work of Sabom (1980; Sabom and Kreutziger, 1978, reprinted in this book) and Ring (1980) has rightly stressed the importance of prospective research. Respondents were selected on the basis of undergoing a near-death event, not necessarily a near-death experience. Both researchers found that over 40 percent of the patients who had undergone near-death events had the experience we are trying to explain. This seems to show that the NDE is a common clinical occurrence. However, this may be a hasty conclusion. Patients who have had an unusual experience when on the verge of death might be more likely to respond to a questionnaire than patients not having had such an experience, thus biasing the sample. A truly prospective investigation of NDEs would have to take place within a given hospital where all resuscitated patients were asked, as a part of the routine examination, whether or not they recalled any unusual experiences.

Special Problems in Trying to Assess NDEs

Near-death phenomena are not easy to assess impartially. One reason is the emotional reactions they arouse. On the one hand, people disposed to believe in life after death may be inclined toward credulity. On the other hand, those disposed to equate belief in survival with outmoded superstition might be prone to avoid dealing with the more challenging features of NDEs. Another reason is intellectual. The prevailing scientific orthodoxy tends in one way or another to identify human beings with their physical organisms; this, in effect, logically rules out any meaningful concept of "survival" after death. In short, the survival hypothesis, which is one possible explanation of NDEs, appears to be peculiarly resistant to rational and scientific investigation.

Requirements for an Adequate
Scientific Theory of NDEs

The first requirement for any scientific theory or hypothesis is that it be consistent with all aspects of the phenomena being studied. But consistency by itself is not enough; more than one hypothesis may be consistent with the phenomena. It is also necessary to show that competing hypotheses don't work. Further, the theory must be consistent with the total system of knowledge. If this consistency is not forthcoming, large-scale revisions in this system may be necessary. Finally, an adequate theory should enable us to predict new features and ramifications of the *explicanda*. Given these requirements, I don't think we know enough about near-death phenomena to provide a decisive theory or explanation. At most, we can take the first step and try to see whether some of the explanations that have already been proposed are consistent with the reported phenomena.

EXPLANATIONS OF NEAR-DEATH EXPERIENCES

The Bipolar Model of Osis and Haraldsson

Using information from a pilot study (Osis, 1961), and other sources, Osis and Haraldsson constructed a model to predict patterns in deathbed phenomena; this model is a "bipolar" one which contrasts two mutually exclusive hypotheses: survival and destruction. They then compared these two poles of explanation with relevant patterns in the findings on deathbed visions from their cross-cultural surveys of deathbed phenomena in the United States and India (Osis and Haraldsson, 1977a, 1977b). The patterns, involved had to do with the source and content of the visions, the influence on them of various medical and psychological factors, and their variability of content across individuals and cultures. Consider, for example, the influence of hallucinogenic factors; on the assumption of the survival hypothesis, the authors predict that drugs known to cause hallucinations will not increase the frequency of survival-related visions, nor will other states in which contact with reality is weakened or absent. They also predict on the survival hypothesis that conditions known to be incompatible with the occurrence of ESP will decrease the frequency of such visions. Regarding this point, for instance, the authors found that the majority of the reported deathbed hallucinations were visual and of short duration—which is the case in most spontaneous ESP experiences. (Pathological hallucinations tend to be auditory.) And finally, they found that, unlike the case of pathological hallucinations, there was little variability in the content of deathbed visions across individuals and cultures, again a finding compatible with the survival hypothesis. The authors conclude that overall the "central tendencies" of their data are consistent with the survival hypothesis of near-death experiences as they formulated it in their bipolar model (Osis and Haraldsson, 1977a, p. 258).

Let us now look at several reductionistic explanations of near-death experiences, some of them engendered by criticisms of the Osis-Haraldsson work, and then proceed to a discussion of a nonreductionistic Jungian approach and the survival hypothesis in an effort to understand these experiences.

Medical Factors

Drugs and Sensory Deprivation. The parapsychologist John Palmer (1978) has criticized the work of Osis and Haraldsson (1977a), who in turn provided a lengthy rejoinder (1978). The main thrust of Palmer's remarks is that certain baseline data are lacking in the study which invalidate the major conclusions, e.g., that medical factors such as drugs did not significantly influence the deathbed apparitions. Osis and Haraldsson contend that they did take the relevant information into account in interpreting their data, and that this information was derived from medical literature and the judgments of medically trained respondents. A major point made by Osis and Haraldsson in their response to Palmer is that the counter-survival explanation has to fit a special *type* of apparition—namely, the survival-related apparition. One cannot explain away deathbed visions simply by saying that drugs produce hallucinations; you must show that the kinds of hallucinations typically produced by drugs fit the pattern of hallucinations occurring in the deathbed scenario. But this is no easy matter, for typical drug-produced hallucinations are not at all like typical near-death hallucinations.

Palmer points out (p. 394) that sensory deprivation and stress are known to facilitate hallucinations. This is true. In a study of the psychological aspects of cardiovascular disease, for example, Reiser and Bakst (1975, p. 637) speak of the "simultaneous sensory overstimulation and monotony" prevailing in the hospital recovery room or intensive care unit—conditions conducive to hallucinatory experiences. Three factors, however, clearly differentiate such hospital-induced hallucinations from NDEs. First, the former usually take place hours or days after the close brush with death, while the latter are reported by the patient as having occurred during the resuscitation procedures. Second, the postoperative effects in the first group of patients consist largely of "confusion, disorientation, and misperceptions," while the hallucinations of the ND experients are often reported as vivid, detailed, and accompanied by feelings of joy. And finally, Kornfeld and Zimberg (1965) describe the behavior of patients in the first group who "go berserk" and try to flee from the medical attendants; this type of behavior contrasts sharply with the frequently reported behavior of NDE patients who become angry when they are restored to normal consciousness.

Cerebral Anoxia and Temporal Lobe Seizures. In a review of Osis and Haraldsson's (1977b) *At the Hour of Death,* James F. McHarg (1978), a British psychiatrist, criticized the authors for failing to consider the "most important" (p. 886) explanation for their ND findings: cerebral anoxia (oxygen shortage in brain metabolism). Osis and Haraldsson (1979) reply that the main behavioral manifestations of cerebral anoxia are anxiety, disorientation, and distortions of perception. These are poor matches for the ND syndrome. Further, there are reports (in Audette, 1979) of the extensive but hitherto unpublished work of Schoonmaker, a Denver cardiologist, who found cases of typical near-death experience in which cerebral anoxia was definitely ruled out as a relevant factor.

McHarg also considers temporal lobe paroxysms (epileptic seizures) and cites three examples from his current clinical work. McHarg adds an important point: "A paranormal basis for the *content* of deathbed visions is not invalidated, however, by a medical reason for their mere occurrence" (p. 886). But McHarg goes on to suggest that what Osis and Haraldsson take to be survival-related features of deathbed visions—e.g., seeing apparitions of the dead with a take-away purpose and feeling religious elation—are "rather *typical* [emphasis mine] of temporal lobe paroxysms." This, however, seems to me an unverified exaggeration. There are actually a variety of epilepsies with varied symptomatology. Temporal lobe seizures are commonly displayed in bizarre, explosive episodes (Elliot, 1966); for example, a patient urinated into a fireplace, another climbed into a window-display of pastries—unaware of what they were doing. Visual aspects of seizures, unlike those of the classic NDE, consist of "dimness of vision, hemianopia [blindness in half of the visual field], blindness, crude flashes of light" (Elliot, 1966, p. 143). Furthermore, Schoonmaker (see Audette, 1979) is said to have collected to date fifty-five cases in which resuscitated NDE patients displayed flat electroencephalograms, i.e., no brain waves. This clashes with the idea of temporal lobe paroxysms since they consist of deviant patterns of electrical activity in the brain, not the absence of such activity.

The temporal lobe is associated with memory, and seizures in that area often evoke memories. We are reminded of Penfield's (1975) experiments on electro-stimulation of the temporal lobe which evoked vivid memories in epileptic patients. Penfield, however, underlines the mechanical nature of these electro-resuscitations of memories; this, again, contrasts with the meaningful experience of meeting others in a transformative near-death experience.

Finally, what if some NDEs were accompanied by temporal lobe paroxysms? McHarg notes that such brain dysfunctions could conceivably facilitate paranormal experience. Perhaps McHarg's patients—those who were not near death—were catching glimpses of another world. Why must transworld ESP occur, if it does occur, only among those who are near death? There might be other conditions of eruption into the "other" world—natural, spontaneous, or even deliberately inducible.

Religious Expectations

Palmer (1978, p. 395) thinks that dying patients who believe in survival expect to be taken away by apparitions; hence their hallucinations may be generated by their expectations. But what about the "no-consent" cases, in which the patient departs under protest? This seems to indicate an external agency. And there are also cases where the patient has no religious beliefs and expects nothing in particular. On the whole, the empirical findings across the board so far indicate that religious beliefs influence the interpretation, not the content, of experiences of this nature.

Even more problematic is Palmer's assumption that believers expect a benign reception committee to greet them at the time of death. Actually, there is plenty of evidence from religious phenomenology indicating less sanguine anticipations. Christian and Hindu iconography and mythology are replete with intimations of post-mortem horrors; in both traditions there are many paintings, illustrated manuscripts, and icons which depict the moment of death as a perilous passage, a frightful encounter with the forces of good and evil. From a psychological point of view, religion seems to encourage attitudes of collective guilt, enshrined in such doctrines as Original Sin. Certainly the ancient Greek *Hades* or the Babylonian *Kurniga* (land of no return) did not suggest any blithe expectations. According to the *Tibetan Book of the Dead* (Evans-Wentz, 1957), there is—as Moody, Ring, and others have found—a Being of Light awaiting us at death; but the religious Being of Light is awe-inspiring, terrifying, and most of us cannot bear the thought of facing it.

The Epicureans of Graeco-Roman antiquity happily embraced a form of materialism whose chief charm was a promise of extinction after death. For the Epicureans this seemed an improvement over the anticipated terrors of the after-world. One could indeed make a good case for an irrational basis to the rise of modern materialism as a form of flight from the tyranny of priests and their infernal visions of an after-life. The empirical picture, by and large, is more humane; happily, it clashes with the paranoid propensities of the religious imagination. I want to bring this point out because certain explanations of ND phenomena arouse resistance among the more rigidly rational types of modern man. There are historico-psychological reasons for this defensive armoring against everything "occult," "spiritual," or "supernatural."

Depersonalization

In one of their several papers on near-death experiences, Noyes and Kletti (1976) suggest a psychologically reductionistic explanation of the phenomena: that they are expressions of the "depersonalization syndrome" (feelings of unreality, emotional detachment, slowing of time, etc.). Let me begin with a comment on the title of this paper: "Depersonalization in the Face of Life-Threatening Danger: A Description." This seems to indicate that the authors did not set out to describe, but rather—as shown by the term "depersonalization" in the title—to place an interpretation on the phenomena. "Depersonalization" is hardly a descriptive term. The authors appear to have ruled out at the start any but a reductionistic explanation. However, this explanation is forced; depersonalization does not adequately characterize near-death phenomena. The main difficulty is that the two types of experience have opposite affects: depersonalization tends toward a flattening affect and shriveling mental capacities. It is essentially a negative phenomenon. In NDEs, on the other hand, we observe an opposite tendency toward heightened affect, expanded awareness, and a sense of profound and lasting significance.

In connection with one of their cases, Noyes and Kletti (1976) describe what they call the feeling of unreality. The subject reported that as she went deeper, reality vanished and visions, soft lights and an extreme feeling of calm acceptance passed over me like waves....I was stronger because of being more whole, because I was no longer me as I had once known myself. I had a feeling of becoming part of a greater whole....[p. 22]

The authors are too hasty in forcing this vanishing of reality into the pathological slot of the depersonalization syndrome. Their tacit assumption seems to be that any deviation from standard, everyday reality must be pathological. The possibility that what was involved was the loss of only one sense of reality, and that another sense of reality was emerging does not seem to occur to Noyes and Kletti. The experience doesn't describe a loss in an exclusively negative sense; the loss also involved a gain, an opening into a larger reality. In fact, the enlarged sense of reality seems to have been in part a function of the loss of personal identity in the narrow sense. The subject seems not to have been *de*personalized, but—more accurately—*trans*personalized.

Schizoid Defense

Several psychologists have discussed the way the fear of death gives rise to defensive belief-systems involving the notion of a soul distinct and separable from the body, and able to survive death. According to this way of thinking, belief in an immortal principle of man is seen as a disguised alienation from the body—a schizoid solution to the brutal problems of being human. R.D. Laing (1965) is no reductionist, but he has provided trenchant descriptions of the "unembodied self": there is, according to Laing, an existential process whereby a person, in the face of the oppression and terrors of existence, retreats to his inner self and creates a private citadel safe from the disasters of the external world. Could this help us to explain near-death experiences? Laing writes: "In this position the individual experiences his self as being more or less divorced or detached from his body. The body is felt more as one object among others in the world than as the core of the individual's own being" (p. 69). This alienation from the body, which Laing sees as a strategy of desperation, tends to produce the schizoid personality. Schizophrenia, according to Laing, is only an extreme development of this basic defense strategy.

The schizoid tendency would be aggravated in a near-death crisis—and it is true that reports of NDEs are replete with accounts of alterations of the patient's body image such as those Laing describes. But in his account of the schizoid process everything culminates in sensations of inner deadness leading to a need to re-establish contact with the external world. This is the reverse of the near-death process, where we typically observe an enlivening of affect along with a readiness to let go of the external world.

Narcissism, Denial of Death, and Freudian Reductionism

Few people have written more searchingly on the denial of death than the psychoanalyst, Otto Rank. In his collection of essays, *The Double,* Rank (1971) examines the widespread phenomenon of the double as it appears in literature, folklore, and anthropology. The empirical cases that Rank looks at—e.g., those of de Maupassant and Goethe—are instances of autoscopy. In these, the percipient sees an apparition of himself in outer space. This, of course, is unlike the typical out-of-body experience associated with a near-death crisis in which the perceiving consciousness seems to be located outside the body. Nevertheless, Rank generalizes from the autoscopic phenomena and chooses to see all constructs "of soul, higher worlds, and immortality" as projections of the narcissistic ego in the face of the "increasing reality-experience of man, who does not want to admit that death is everlasting annihilation" (p. 84). Rank is uncompromising in his Freudian reductionist judgment: "The idea of death therefore is denied by a duplication of the self incorporated in the shadow or in the reflected image." This makes short shrift of the highest human dreams. It is an outlook which inverts the classic Platonic formula: Plato's image-sensory world is now the really real world and the realm of ideas and ideals are reduced to images and shadows. Thanks to his commitment to Freudian dogma, Rank can speak confidently of "increasing reality-experience" as if the only real experiences were definable in terms of a single reality principle.

But there are two lines of reasoning that do not tally with Rank's conclusions. First, he describes the personality characteristics of those who generate "double" phenomena; they seem to be narcissists—persons with pathological fixations on themselves. If this is so, then "double" phenomena ought to be proportional to narcissistic behaviors. This is not an obviously true proposition. But we might be able to formulate such a claim in a testable way—for example, we could predict that persons who have the most gratifying NDEs also display a significant frequency of narcissistic traits. At the moment, however, there is no evidence in support of such a relationship.

The second difficulty with Freudian reductionism is the veridical psi-component sometimes found in OBEs and NDEs. The psychiatrist Jan Ehrenwald (1978) follows Rank in claiming that OBEs "exhibit an assorted set of defenses and rationalizations aimed at warding off anxiety originating from the breakdown of the body image, from the threatening split or disorganization of the ego, and, in the last analysis, from the fear of death as a universal experience" (p. 161). Unlike Rank, however, Ehrenwald has thought and written a great deal about psi. He admits that some OBEs (and no doubt some NDEs) contain veridical information that strains the wish-fulfilling hypothesis; but this is not enough to persuade him that OBEs are not fundamentally delusive and the product of denial of death. As far as I can see, however, this is little more than the expression of a metaphysical dogma. After all, it is hard to see why, if an experience is merely a subjective wish-fulfillment, it should contain any verifiable, objective information. Moreover, many persons who have had OBEs report that their lives were significantly and permanently changed by these experiences (see, e.g., Osis and McCormack, 1978); such changes are not what we would expect to result from narcissistic illusions. And there is still another point about OBEs which is at odds with the Freudian interpretation. There are numerous cases in which the experient becomes frightened after finding himself out of the body; the fear of death results from the experience itself and causes its sudden termination. Thus the fear of death seems to inhibit the experience rather than give rise to it.

The Birth Experience

According to Stanislav Grof, a researcher into the therapeutic and theoretical implications of psychoactive chemicals, subjects under the influence of LSD often relive aspects of the birth process (Grof and Halifax, 1977). The contention—quite plausible, especially in the light of Penfield's (1975) work on the neuro-electrical activation of memories—is that under special circumstances we may re-experience the agony of expulsion from the amniotic sac of "oceanic bliss" into the world of individual existence. For Grof these traumatic birth memories have important therapeutic implications. He is not, however, a Freudian reductionist; on the contrary, he has used nonspecific chemical amplifiers of consciousness to enrich and enlarge the cartography of inner space.

Based on Grof's observations, the astronomer Carl Sagan (1979) suggests an intriguing explanation of near-death experiences in his popular tour of the wonderland of modern science, *Broca's Brain.* He poses the problem effectively: "How could it be that people of all ages, cultures and eschatological predispositions have the *same sort* of near-death experience?" (p. 302). Sagan speculates that the basis of near-death and mystical experiences is somehow "wired-in" (note the characteristic mechanical type of metaphor) to the physiology of the human organism, and that drugs or other types of mechanism might trigger and thus reactivate these experiences in the form of vivid hallucinations. Out-of-body experiences would be affective replays of ejection from the womb at birth. The tunnel effect reported so frequently in NDEs might represent a flashback to the process of exiting through the "tunnel" of the vagina. (It might, of course, as well be seen as the psychic equivalent of the process of exiting from the present dying body.) Sagan writes:

> Every human being, without exception, has already shared an experience like that of those travellers who return from the land of death: the sensation of flight, the emergence from darkness into light; an experience in which, at least sometimes, a heroic figure can be dimly perceived, bathed in radiance and glory. There is only one common experience that matches this description. It is called birth. [P. 304]

Sagan calls attention in this quotation to three important ideas. One is that we seem to be dealing with a basic mechanism of psychophysiology. The second is that there is a fundamental analogy between the birth process and the death process. And third is that NDEs and mystical experiences are somehow structurally related.

However, the difficulty arises in seeing the NDE as nothing but an illusory psychophysiological reflex. At least we would require some evidence in support of the hypothesis; for instance, if Sagan is right, then people who had bad births—difficulties in the process of exiting through the birth canal, etc.—should not have benign near-death experiences. (And would those who come into the world by way of caesarean section be immune to NDEs?) Yet even if such connections were established, nothing would follow concerning the "reality" of near-death episodes. Other factors need to be taken into consideration, such as the occurrence of veridical psi components. Further, the essential structures of birth and death experiences differ in this way: birth moves from "amniotic bliss" to expulsion into the traumatic light. The pattern in the near-death process is the reverse: we begin with the pain and shock of the dying process, and then proceed to experience a light which, however, is uniformly said to be warm, loving, and gentle. If the near-death experience is a flashback and replica of the birth experience, why this inconsistency? The forms of the two processes are not analogous, as we would expect if one were a flashback of the other. They seem in fact to be the reverse of each other: being born into this world is painful and dying out of it seems to be pleasant. It is clear that we are not yet any closer to an adequate explanation of near-death experiences.

A NONREDUCTIONISTIC JUNGIAN APPROACH TO NEAR-DEATH EXPERIENCES

Grof, from whom Sagan borrowed to formulate his hypothesis about NDEs, is a phenomenologist with Jungian leanings. Data emerging from psychedelic research led him to validate Jung's concept of archetypes and their relation to the stream of our personal consciousness. Grof, like Jung, was clearly not disposed to reducing them to mere physiological epiphenomena. I would like to propose a possible Jungian explanation of near-death experiences. At the same time, I believe that this approach will have to be supplemented by findings from parapsychology.

The Archetype of Death

I shall make use of two assumptions from the field of Jungian analytical psychology. The first assumption is that certain collective psychic structures—forms, ideas, archetypes, empirically substantiated by data from dreams and mythology—in some logically prior way exist, free from the limits of space and time. The archetypes represent the point of intersection between personal time and timeless transpersonal being. Jung (1968) himself put it this way:

> The deepest we can reach in our exploration of the unconscious mind is the layer where man is no longer a distinct individual, but where his mind widens out and merges into the mind of mankind—not the conscious mind, but the unconscious mind of mankind, where we are all the same. [P. 46]

The second assumption is that the archetypes function to assist the growth and evolution of the personality. Jung calls this process "individuation." The archetypes come into play especially during mental emergencies, as automatic responses to crises of individuation. Jung (1971, p. 38) also stresses what he calls archetypes of transformation, which involve "typical situations, places, ways and means, that symbolize the kind of transformation in question." One other immediately relevant thing to note is the ineffable, paradoxical, and numinous nature of the archetypes.

Research on near-death experiences may be uncovering data which empirically support the hypothesis of an "Idea" or "Archetype of Death"—a collective psychic structure whose function is to assist a human personality during a major crisis of individuation. According to Jungian theory, such an archetype would represent and contain the racial memory and wisdom of mankind. The collective experience of the human race has come up with this as the best possible way to die. The archetype is a paradigm—an old Platonic term—for how to die. It is optimally functional for dying in the same way the lung through evolution has become optimally functional for breathing. Near-death phenomena point toward an archetype or paradigm for a healthy death—a somewhat paradoxical expression, I admit.

The advantage of this explanation is that it saves the important subjective phenomena: the experience of ineffable unity, transcendental elation, and so forth. For, as Jung claims, the archetypes are merging phenomena with numinous overtones. It also accounts for the transformative effects of NDEs, which seem to involve release from the limitations of ordinary, space-time bound, individual existence. Yet there remain two thorny problems for the hypothesis of a death archetype. First, what is the fate of personal consciousness in this archetypal transformation of death? Second, what are we to make of the psi components of NDEs? The genuine paranormal effects obviously occur in a specifiable space-time framework and seem to involve awareness of particular deceased individuals.

According to the theory of archetypes, superpersonal structures "survive" death partly because they never undergo birth the way individual bodies do. Before John Jones was, the archetypes are. But what happens (in this Platonic-Jungian atemporal world) to the personal consciousness of John Jones? Some of the testimony from near-death cases indicates that the unique personality survives, for what the experients often claim they "see" are the apparitions of recognizable, unique beings. Of course, this is not all; other things are also "seen," sensed as amorphous presences, or otherwise "perceived" as mythic forms. In the world glimpsed by dying patients, personal and transpersonal elements apparently co-exist. The near-death experience, like the Jungian archetype, is full of paradox. It strains the limits of our normal conceptual apparatus, as if it would in some way both unite and dissolve opposites.

The facts seem to support a paradoxical explanation of the fate of the individual. The description from Noyes and Kletti (1976) that I quoted above bears repeating: "I was no longer *me* as I had once known myself. I had a feeling of becoming part of a greater whole." This speaks of a transformation of personal identity. There are different ways of describing this fundamental experience. Some call it the highest quest of the mystic, others regression to the magical omnipotence of primary narcissism. How shall we decide which interpretation to place upon this basic phenomenon of transcendence? This brings us once again to the paranormal factor in NDEs.

The Psi Component

The reductionist has neat and coherent schemes for digesting the dreams of artists and the visions of mystics and dying persons. But it is no easy matter for them to swallow such puzzling fish as ESP and PK. It is the psi component in near-death experiences that stands squarely in the way of reducing them to being mere illusions.

But having said this, we must also consider the explanation offered by parapsychological reductionists. They would claim that if we combine the known paranormal powers of embodied minds with a basically Freudian metaphysics, we can account for the near-death phenomena and still reject the survival hypothesis. Suppose a dying patient experiences a veridical apparition of a relative who died before the patient was born, precognizes in detail some unusual future event, or provides a verifiable report of being out of the body. Why, these parapsychologists ask, can't we say that this is merely an example of the patient's psi operating in the service of a regressive tendency toward wish-fulfillment? In fact, there is hardly anything, no matter how remote from "ordinary" reality, that they do not ascribe to the supposed infinite psi-potential of the living human being. This "super-ESP" hypothesis (Gauld, 1961), as it is called, has been aptly characterized by Osis (1979) as "that strange invention which shies like a mouse from being tested in the laboratory but, in rampant speculations, acts like a ferocious lion devouring the survival evidence" (p. 31).

Moreover, as other parapsychologists have argued, if such extraordinary paranormal abilities exist in human beings, then it seems plausible to take the next step and consider the possibility of survival. In short, the super-ESP hypothesis is self-canceling, for the more effectively it argues for fantastic powers of the living mind, the less implausible—in fact, the more probable—it seems that there is an element of human personality capable of surviving after death.

THE SURVIVAL HYPOTHESIS

The immediate attraction of the survival hypothesis is its consistency with the beliefs of almost all those who have had the classic near-death experience. Ring (1980), for example, found a "huge effect" here. Although those having the experience were found to be less inclined to believe in survival to start with, as compared to nonexperiencers, they were much more likely to believe in it afterwards. Thus, as Ring points out, it is not merely "coming close to death that tends to convince one that there is life after death; it is...the experience itself that proves decisive. The testimony here is unambiguous" (p. 169). Of course, since the claims of these experients, particularly those about the nature of the afterworld, are not publicly verifiable, we cannot consider them as direct evidence for survival. But a mass of such accounts with congruent claims must, after a critical point, begin to count as a special consensus. Is it possible that those who come closer to experiencing death know by acquaintance more about death than the rest of us do?

Needless to say, this will not do for the skeptic. Belief in life after death is unpopular among most intellectuals today. One reason for this is that there are supposedly good a priori arguments against the conceivability of survival. An excellent discussion of this problem from a philosophical point of view is offered by H.D. Lewis (1978) in *Persons and Life After Death*. The prevailing conception of the person nowadays derives from physicalism, the ruling philosophy that sees everything mental as ultimately reducible to physical states. Yet the major tendency of parapsychological research is to upset the pretensions of physicalism. Indeed, some able persons have argued the case for the impossibility of reducing psi phenomena to physical principles (see, for example, Beloff, 1980). This is a problem that requires full discussion. I will only remark here that the more unlikely it becomes that psi can be explained in terms of physical principles, the more intrinsically plausible the survival hypothesis becomes.

An evaluation of the survivalist explanation of near-death phenomena demands a full account of other types of evidence for survival, such as mediumistic communications, veridical apparitions of the deceased, and reincarnation memories. Explaining NDEs is obviously a large undertaking. The most that can be said now is that they cannot be adequately accounted for by any of the reductionist theories, but that to invoke either Jungian or outright survival hypotheses would be premature. To embrace such non-reductionistic explanations is to commit oneself to far-reaching revisions of the general nature of things. One desires more solid ground from which to make such transcendental leaps. In the light of the facts, one is entitled to abstain from final judgment and rest in the skeptical attitude—but this means with regard to the pronouncements of physicalism as well as to the claims of survivalists. One is rendered free—in a Jamesian, pragmatic way—to accept the survival hypothesis, for such a belief is consistent with near-death phenomena. But the great question of who we are and what our fate is after death is still open. We may be on the threshold of new discoveries. Whether we advance or whether we stagnate in indifference will depend on the courage and collaboration of many, both hard-headed scientists and students of the humanities.

Notes

1. This example is taken from a tape recording of a lecture given by Dr. Sabom at the Psychical Research Foundation (Sabom, 1980; see also Sabom and Kreutziger, 1978).

References

Audette, J.R. 1979. "Denver Cardiologist Discloses Findings After 18 Years of Near-Death Research." *Anabiosis* 1:1-2.

————. 1982. "Historical Perspectives on Near-Death Episodes and Experiences." In C. Lundahl (Comp.), *A Collection of Near-Death Research Readings.* Chicago: Nelson-Hall.

Barrett. W.F., 1926. *Death-Bed Visions.* London: Methuen.

Beloff, J. 1980. "Could There Be a Physical Explanation for Psi?" *Journal of the Society for Psychical Research* 50:263-72.

Bozzano, E. 1906. "Apparitions of Deceased Persons at Death-Beds." *Annals of Psychical Science,* pp. 67-100.

————. 1923. *Phenomenes Psychiquies au Moment de la Mort.* Paris: Nicholas Renault.

————. 1948. *Dei Fenomeni di Telecinesia in Rapporto con Eventi di Morte.* Verona: Casa Editrice Europa.

Crookall, R. 1965. *Intimations of Immortality.* Exeter, England: James Clarke.

Ehrenwald, J. 1978. *The ESP Experience.* New York: Basic Books.

Elliot, F.A. 1966. *Clinical Neurology.* Philadelphia and London: Saunders.

Evans-Wentz, W.Y. (Ed.). 1957. *The Tibetan Book of the Dead.* 3rd ed. London: Oxford University Press.

Gauld, A. 1961. "The Super-ESP Hypothesis." *Proceedings of the Society for Psychical Research* 53:226-46.

Grof, S., and J. Halifax. 1977. *The Human Encounter with Death.* New York: Dutton.

Grosso, M. 1979. "Near-Death Experience and the Eleusinian Mysteries." Paper presented at Founder's Day, Psychical Research Foundation, April.

Honorton, C. 1977. "Psi and Internal Attention States." In B.B. Wolman (Ed.), *Handbook of Parapsychology.* New York: Van Nostrand Reinhold.

Hyslop, J.H. 1908. *Psychical Research and the Resurrection.* Boston: Small, Maynard.

Jung, C.G. 1968. *Analytical Psychology: Its Theory and Practice.* New York: Random House.

————. 1971. *The Archetypes of the Collective Unconscious.* Princeton, N.J.: Princeton University Press.

Kornfeld, D.S., and S. Zimberg. 1965. "Psychiatric Complications of Open-Heart Surgery." *New England Journal of Medicine* 273:287-92.

Laing, R.D. 1965. *The Divided Self.* Baltimore: Pelican Books.

Lewis, H.D. 1978. *Persons and Life After Death.* New York: Harper and Row.

Lundahl, C.R. (Comp.). 1982. *A Collection of Near-Death Research Readings.* Chicago: Nelson-Hall.

McHarg, J.F. 1978. Review of *At the Hour of Death* by K. Osis and E. Haraldsson. *Journal of the Society for Psychical Research* 49:885-87; see also 1979, 50:128-29, for further discussion.

Moody, R.A., Jr. 1975. *Life After Life.* Atlanta: Mockingbird Books.

———. 1977. *Reflections on Life After Life.* New York: Bantam Books.

Noyes, R. 1971. "Dying and Mystical Consciousness." *Journal of Thanatology* 1:25-41.

Noyes, R. and R. Kletti. 1976. "Depersonalization in the Face of Life-Threatening Danger: A Description." *Psychiatry* 39:19-27.

Osis, K. 1961. *Deathbed Observations by Physicians and Nurses.* New York: Parapsychology Foundation.

Osis, K. 1979. "Research on Near-Death Experiences: A New Look." In W.G. Roll (Ed.), *Research in Parapsychology 1978.* Metuchen, N.J.: Scarecrow Press.

Osis, K., and E. Haraldsson. 1977a. "Deathbed Observations by Physicians and Nurses: A Cross-Cultural Survey." *Journal of the American Society for Psychical Research* 71:237-59.

———. 1977b. *At the Hour of Death.* New York: Avon Books.

———. 1978. Correspondence: Reply to Dr. Palmer. *Journal of the American Society for Psychical Research* 72:395-400.

———. 1979. Correspondence: Reply to Dr. McHarg. *Journal of the American Society for Psychical Research* 50:126-28.

Osis, K., and D. McCormick. 1978. "Insiders' View of the OBE." *ASPR Newsletter* 4:18-19.

Palmer, J. 1978. Correspondence: Deathbed Apparitions and the Survival Hypothesis. *Journal of the American Society for Psychical Research* 72:392-95; see also 1979, 73:94-96, for further discussion.

Penfield, W. 1975. *The Mystery of the Mind.* Princeton, N.J.: Princeton University Press.

Rank, O. 1971. *The Double.* Chapel Hill: University of North Carolina Press.

Reiser, M., and H. Bakst. 1975. "Psychodynamic Problems of the Patient with Structural Heart Disease." In *American Handbook of Psychiatry,* Vol. 4. New York: Basic Books.

Rhine, L.E. 1970. *Mind over Matter*. New York: Macmillan.

Ring, K. 1980. *Life at Death: A Scientific Investigation of the Near-Death Experience*. New York: Coward, McCann and Geoghegan.

Rogo, S. 1979. "Research on Deathbed Experiences: Some Contemporary and Historical Perspectives." *Journal of the Academy of Religion and Psychical Research* 2:37-49.

Russell, G.W. 1965. *The Candle of Vision*. Wheaton, Ill.: Quest.

Sabom, M.B. 1980. "Near-Death Experiences: A Medical Perspective." Paper presented at Founder's Day, Psychical Research Foundation, May.

Sabom, M.B., and S.A. Kreutziger. 1978. "Physicians Evaluate the Near-Death Experience." *Theta* 6 (4):1-6.

Sagan, C. 1979. *Broca's Brain*. New York: Random House.

Sidgwick, H., and Committee. 1894. "Report on the Census of Hallucinations." *Proceedings of the Society for Psychical Reserch* 10:25-422.

PART FIVE

Directions in Near-Death Research

13

Directions in Near-Death Research

Craig R. Lundahl

IN THE PAST DECADE, RESEARCH interest in a phenomenon known as the near-death experience has greatly increased, primarily as a result of Moody's study of 150 cases of people who experienced apparent clinical death or a near-fatal encounter with death (1975). This field of scientific research has been labeled *circumthanatology*—the scientific study of near-death. Since that original study, medical and behavioral scientific work on the near-death experience has proceeded at an increasing rate. Published reports of over three thousand documented cases of near-death experiences in conjunction with near-death episodes justify the assertion that the near-death experience is an authentic phenomenon.

The beginnings of circumthanatology were characterized by the collection and description of the raw data on the near-death experience. More recently, there has been an effort to organize the accumulated knowledge of the field into concepts, generalizations, and theories. A professional organization, the Association for the Scientific Study of Near-Death Phenomena, was established in 1979.

NEW DEVELOPMENTS IN STUDY TECHNIQUES

Near-death research has used a variety of techniques, and the subject matter has been approached from a variety of viewpoints—

Lundahl, C.R. 1981. "Directions in Near-Death Research." *Death Education* 5:135-42.

reflecting an assumption that no single point of view nor research methodology can encompass total reality. Two techniques are now being used for the first time to attempt to verify the near-death experience. The first, employed by Osis and McCormick (1979), suggests that the human personality can exist apart from the physical body. For many years, there have been reports of people who claim to have the ability to separate from their physical bodies. Osis and McCormick selected such a person for their experiment. During the experiment, the person was requested to lie down and allow his personality to leave his physical body and go into an eighteen-inch chamber or box. This chamber was composed of two layers of steel sheeting that provided electromagnetic shielding and electrical shielding and was located six doors away from the subject's physical body. A device was used to display a random array of pictures, which the subject was asked to identify from a viewing window within the chamber. Osis and McCormick also used a polygraph attached to strain gauges connected to suspended sensor plates to register any kinetic effects in the chamber where the subject's personality or consciousness was reportedly located during the experiment. Osis and McCormick found that the polygraph activation level was significantly higher when the subject was identifying the pictures from the viewing window in the chamber, suggesting that the personality or consciousness can exist apart from the physical body. The results of this experiment, although very tentative, can, along with future experiments, help us clarify and better understand the out-of-the-body phase of the near-death experience.

Sabom is attempting to verify the out-of-the-body phase of the near-death experience using another technique—that of gathering specific information on the resuscitative events taking place when a person in a hospital setting has been rendered unconscious at the moment of physical near-death. This information is being collected from medical records and from the patient, the attending hospital staff, and the attending family members, independently of each other. Comparisons are made between the resuscitative events described by the subject in the out-of-the-body experience and the actual situation described by those physically present at the time. Sabom's preliminary findings show remarkable similarities between the two sets of descriptive data. He has observed that sometimes objects and events outside the unconscious person's physical visual field are accurately described in visual detail. Furthermore, the exact sequence of resuscitative measures is also described as if the episode had indeed been witnessed from a detached position. Thus far, the out-of-the-body perceptions related by the subjects closely parallel objective reality.

MAJOR DIRECTIONS IN THE FIELD

Scientific Investigations of Near-Death Experiences

There are a growing number of scientifically derived studies in the field. These studies differ from earlier exploratory and descriptive studies in their enlarged scope and in their attempts to gather data in a much more systematic way. The major objectives of these replication studies are to examine the relationships between variables and to substantiate the prior findings of near-death research.

Soon to be released will be the detailed findings of two recent studies conducted by Ring and Sabom. Ring's study will report the findings of formal interviews with 102 people who survived physical near-death. Sabom's study will report data from interviews of 107 people surviving near-death. His study includes sociologic and demographic data as well as the medical details of each near-death episode.

The report of another study, by Schoonmaker (Audette, 1979), is anxiously awaited by many in the field. Schoonmaker has analyzed 2,300 cases of people experiencing near-death episodes (which may or may not contain near-death experiences) in a Denver, Colorado, hospital since 1961. Three unique features of Schoonmaker's work are: (a) the length of his study—nineteen years, (b) the large number of documented near-death experiences (contained in the near-death episodes)—1,400, and (c) the detailed physiological data recorded for most of the cases. Early indications are that Schoonmaker's data substantiate the findings from earlier exploratory and descriptive studies.

Still another research undertaking by investigators John R. Audette, Dean R. Bordeaux, John R. Day, and Michael Gulley is in progress in Peoria, Illinois. The aim of this research involving the Methodist Medical Center and the Saint Francis Hospital-Medical Center is to conduct a systematic investigation so structured as to remedy the shortcomings of earlier investigations. These investigators intend to collect a minimum of 250 concurrently reported cases of near-death episodes from a sample of four distinct population groups. They hope to examine every conceivably important variable in the near-death experience. Results of this study should be available in the near future.

Postmortem Survival

A second movement in research in circumthanatology is the examination of the question of post-mortem survival. Stevenson and Greyson (1979) have criticized investigators of near-death for ignoring completely the question of whether or not there is survival after death. They point out that the evidence available is far from conclusive on the question of survival after death but that it is also far from deserving the neglect it has received from most scientists. In a recent article they attempt to build a case for directing further inquiries into near-death experiences toward the question of survival.

The classic study of deathbed observations by Osis and Haraldsson (1977) is one of the few studies that deal with the issue of survival after death. These researchers have concluded that the central tendencies of their data support the afterlife hypothesis. They add, however, that the issue of survival after death cannot be assessed solely on the basis of experiences of dying patients, as in their study. Rather, the entire range of other phenomena suggestive of an afterlife, such as out-of-the-body experiences, reincarnation memories, apparitions perceived, and certain kinds of mediumistic communications should be examined.

It seems that the central controversy evolving around this movement pertains to the quesiton of what constitutes evidence of a post-death existence and whether or not the question of such existence can be investigated with our present scientific techniques. Some (Noyes et al., 1977; Ehrenwald, 1974; Lukianowicz, 1958) have already explained away the near-death experience as merely an emotional reaction to the prospect of imminent death, as a defense mechanism to reduce the fear of death, or as an extrasensory perception. Still another investigator, Sabom (1980), believes that, before we can look at the question of life after death, we first must try to determine if the mind can survive apart from the brain or whether we are really looking at evidence for some form of extrasensory perception. Yet, in the opinion of others, such as Ring (1980), individual consciousness may indeed persist after physical death, but even a million amply documented near-death experiences will not prove it. Moody (1979) also finds no justification for viewing near-death experiences as evidence for life after death. It appears that most of the researchers in the field are studying near-death experiences for their own sake irrespective of their implications for the possibilities of the survival of the personality after the death of the physical body.

Clinical Applications of Near-Death Research

Another movement gaining momentum in near-death research is practical application of the findings of near-death research. Among those calling for the clinical application of near-death research findings are Moody, Katz, and Ring.

Moody (1979, p. 6) thinks the most important clinical implication of the work on the near-death experience is that it places those in the fields of medicine and religion in the position of being able "to reassure survivors of close calls with death that they are not alone, that their experiences are relatively common among people in this situation, and that such experiences tend to have remarkably similar forms." What is called for, according to Moody, "is not the application of a diagnostic label, but rather, a sympathetic exploration with the patient of what exactly seemed to him to be happening, allowing him to express his feelings and emotions without having a sense of being adversely judged." A recent study shows that the near-death experience is a clinical event with significant implications for the medical patient and needs to be recognized and understood by health care professionals who care for these patients. Such recognition and understanding, according to this study, is not yet widespread.

In recent years, the hospice has been developed as an alternative to the hospital for the dying patient. The emphasis of hospice care is on the alleviation of the patient's pain and on meeting the patient's human needs. Katz (1979) thinks that, for the hospice patient to achieve maximal support in dying, the hospice staff must be very sensitive to the transpersonal aspects of dying so they can sympathetically discuss them with the dying patient.

Ring (1979) has proposed the establishment of a facility for the dying where the terminally ill would live while being prepared to die, with full awareness of the reality of death as a passage into another dimension of life. This preparation would have three principal components: (a) the alleviation of pain, (b) the alleviation of fears about death, and (c) the preparation for the death experience. Thus, the proposed program would consist of medical, therapeutic, and educational features combined and blended to facilitate a pain-free and fear-free transition into afterlife. Two other functions of the proposed facility would be to serve as a training institute and as a research facility.

An early attempt to apply the findings of near-death research was in the use of bibliotherapy on suicidal patients. McDonagh (1979) reported that reading passages from Moody's book, *Reflections on Life After Life* (1977), had a positive impact on three suicidal patients. He believes this type of treatment merits further use.

CONCLUSION

The study of the near-death experience is dealing with phenomena the meaning of which is still unclear, and much remains to be done. No one knows what the future holds for this new scientific endeavor. It is certain, though, that near-death research has the potential for significantly contributing to our understanding of the death experience in human life. Its findings could have major consequences for all our lives.

References

Audette, J. 1979. "Denver Cardiologist Discloses Findings After 18 Years of Near-Death Research." *Anabiosis* 1:1-2.

Dobson, M., M.W., Adler, A.E., Tattersfield, et al. 1971. "Attitudes and Long-Term Adjustment of Patients Surviving Cardiac Arrest." *British Medical Journal* 3:207-12.

Druss, R.G. and D.S. Kornfeld, 1967. "The Survivors of Cardiac Arrest: A Psychiatric Study." *JAMA* 201:291-96.

Ehrenwald, J. 1974. "Out-of-the-Body Experiences and the Denial of Death." *Journal of Nervous and Mental Disease* 159:227-33.

Garfield, C.A. 1977. "The Dying Patient's Concern with Life After Death." Paper presented at the American Psychological Association meetings, San Francisco, Ca.

Greyson, B. and I. Stevenson. "Near Death Experiences: Characteristic Features." Unpublished manuscript.

Kalish, R. 1969. "Experiences of Persons Reprieved from Death." In A.H. Kutscher (Ed.), *Death and Bereavement.* Springfield, Ill.: Charles C. Thomas.

Katz, J.M. 1979. "Transpersonal Aspects of Dying in Hospice Patients." Paper presented at the American Psychological Association meetings, New York.

Lukianowicz, N. 1958. "Autoscopic Phenomena." *AMA Archives of Neurology and Psychiatry,* 80:199-220.

Lundahl, C.R. (Comp.). 1982. *A Collection of Near-Death Research Readings.* Chicago: Nelson-Hall.

———. 1979. "Mormon Near-Death Experiences." *Free Inquiry in Creative Sociology* 7:101-4, 107.

McDonagh, J. 1979. "Bibliotherapy with Suicidal Patients." Paper presented at the American Psychological Association meetings, New York.

Moody, R.A., Jr. 1975. *Life After Life.* Covington, Ga.: Mockingbird Books.

———. 1977. *Reflections on Life after Life.* Covington, Ga.: Mockingbird Books.

———. 1979. "Clinical Aspects of Near-Death Experiences." Paper presented at the American Psychological Association meetings, New York.

Noyes, R., P.R. Hoenk, S. Kuperman, et al. 1977. "Depersonalization in Accident Victims and Psychiatric Patients." *Journal of Nervous and Mental Disease* 164:401-7.

Noyes, R. and R. Kletti. 1976. "Depersonalization in the Face of Life-Threatening Danger: A Description." *Psychiatry* 39:19-27.

Osis, K. and E. Haraldsson. 1977. *At the Hour of Death.* New York: Avon Books.

———. 1977. "Deathbed Observations by Physicians and Nurses: A Cross-Cultural Survey." *Journal of the American Society of Psychical Research* 71:237-59.

———, and D. McCormick. 1979. "Kinetic Effects at the Ostensible Location of an OB Projection During Perceptual Testing." Paper presented at the Parapsychological Association 22nd Annual Convention, Moraga, Cal.

Ring, K. 1979. "Psychologist Advocates Establishment of a Center for the Dying Based on Near-Death Research Information." *Anabiosis* 1:7-8.

———. 1979. "Further Studies of the Near-Death Experience." *Theta,* 7:1-3.

———. Forthcoming. "Commentary on the Reality of Death Experiences: A Personal Perspective by Ernst A. Rodin." *Journal of Nervous and Mental Disease.*

————. In press. *Life at Death: A Scientific Investigation of the Near-Death Experience.* New York: Coward, McCann, and Geoghegan.

Rosen, D. 1975. "Suicide Survivors: A Follow-Up Study of Persons Who Survived Jumping from the Golden Gate and San Francisco-Oakland Bay Bridges." *Western Journal of Medicine* 122:289-94.

Sabom, M.B. In press. *Recollections of Death.* New York: Harper and Row.

————. 1979. "The Near-Death Experience: Clinical and Religious Implications." Paper presented at the American Psychological Association meetings, New York.

————, and S.A. Kreutziger. 1977. "The Experience of Near Death." *Death Education* 1:195-203.

————. 1978. "Physicians Evaluate the Near-Death Experience." *Theta* 6:1-6.

————. 1980. Personal communication.

Stevenson, I. and G. Greyson. 1979. "Near-Death Experiences. Relevance to the Question of Survival After Death." *JAMA* 242:265-67.

DATE DUE

JA F4 '85			
NO 18 '85			
GAYLORD			PRINTED IN U.S.A.